Anna Garrett Companies LLC
Asheville, NC
info@drannagarrett.com

Dr. Anna Garrett, author
Rebecca Frederick and Anna Caddell, cover art
Kristi Hedberg, cover photograph

ISBN 978-0-9600583-0-3   Paperback
ISBN 978-0-9600583-1-0   eBook

First Edition

This is a work of nonfiction. Some names and identifying details have been changed.

Table of Contents

Dedication

This book is dedicated to Stephanie,
Jennifer and Caroline.

Author's Note

I'm often asked why I decided to write this book. There are many reasons, but the main inspiration is that I saw a need that was not being filled. Three years ago, I started a group called The Hormone Harmony Club on Facebook (www.drannagarrett.com/hhc). It is a private group where members can ask anything they want about perimenopause and menopause. As the group grew, I began to notice there were huge gaps in what women knew about their bodies and the process of perimenopause. I also discovered that the quality of information about perimenopause was seriously lacking.

For the last three years, I have been writing blogs, making videos, answering questions, and thinking about how best to serve women who are confused, scared and hungry for information. All of that work has become the basis for this book. My goal is to create a new generation of what I call "Savvy Sisters." Savvy Sisters are women who are informed, know how to advocate for themselves with their healthcare team, and refuse to settle for suffering. They are role models for their daughters and granddaughters when it comes to asking for what they need and expecting to get it. I know we have a long way to go, but my hope is that this book will help keep the conversation going and gaining momentum.

The stories I tell throughout this book are true. Names have been changed and some contain an amalgamation of multiple client experiences. They illustrate how vastly different the experiences of women can be. May they bring comfort to those of you who feel alone on this journey. Trust me, you are not.

I've included information about different approaches you can try to improve to your perimenopause experience. Many are lifestyle changes, but there are supplement recommendations as well. If you are considering incorporating supplements, please ask your pharmacist if there are any interactions with other medications you take. It is very important that you do your due diligence to find out if a recommendation made here is appropriate for you. And please remember, nothing in this book should be substituted for your doctor's advice.

My goal is to spread the word through speaking to women's groups and consulting with wellness programs and corporations to create a culture of empathy and caring where women are empowered to speak up and ask for what they need. If you believe my message will resonate with your group or organization and you're interested in having me speak, please contact me at info@drannagarrett.com. I also work with individuals to help them create a midlife roadmap that incorporates hormone balance, genetics, and lifestyle management so they can rock their mojo through midlife and beyond. Schedule a consultation with me at www.drannagarrett.com/lets-talk.

Introduction

If you picked up this book, I'll bet I know something about you. In the back of your mind, you're concerned because you just don't feel like yourself. Maybe it's little things, such as feeling a bit more edgy (to put it nicely) with your partner and kids. Maybe you've gotten to the point where you're afraid to leave your house for the first couple of days of your period because it's so heavy. Or maybe you lie awake night after night, staring at the ceiling, when you'd always been a great sleeper. Whatever it is for you, you want answers and you want to know how to cope.

I remember running to the bookstore when I was first pregnant with my daughter and proudly buying my copy of *What to Expect When You're Expecting*. It has long been the bible of pregnant moms everywhere because of the step-by-step info walking you through your entire pregnancy. No guessing. No wondering if you were normal. What a gift this was for me and my friends!

And here we all are again…twenty years later. But this time, we're dealing with the hormonal issues that arise in midlife and there's no perimenopause bible. Menopause is a natural part of life that ALL women will experience, but the way we experience it can be vastly different. Fifty-seven percent of women will experience one or more symptoms of perimenopause as they transition to menopause. The other 43 percent have irregular periods and nothing more. Lucky ladies! Perimenopause and menopause are talked about only in whispers, although this is beginning to change. Doctors are not well trained in how to manage all of the mind, body, and spirit issues that affect women in midlife, so we are most often left to consult Dr. Google for answers. The problem with this is that there is a plethora of misinformation on the internet.

In my work, I see many women who feel as if their bodies are betraying them. They feel like shells of their once-productive, loving selves, and it breaks my heart. They are desperate to find relief and jump from solution to solution, hoping they'll stumble upon the magic bullet. Perimenopause can last over 10 years, and that is not good news for many women. That's a lot of time to be miserable when help can be had.

Desperation is a bad place to make good decisions from, and it leads women to make unwise choices about who they take advice from. That's what led me to write this book. I am tired of seeing bad information shared as gospel in Facebook groups. I am tired of watching women go blindly through this change. I am tired of perimenopause being talked about as a disease. It is not. It is a perfectly healthy, natural progression of our reproductive years.

Savvy Sisters don't suffer silently. I want this book to be the second talk our mothers should have had with us to give us some kind of clue about what was coming with perimenopause and menopause. I want to drive out fear and bring in hope. I want women to see midlife for what it can be and not the beginning of the end or the expiration of their role as mother and caretaker. I want to create a generation of Savvy Sisters who know exactly what's going on. So, let's get on with it. Start by taking my perimenopause quiz at www.perimenopausequiz.com. Then, take a deep breath and start reading. Your answers are here, and there is nothing to be afraid of.

Chapter 1:
What is THIS Fresh Hell?

Janie is 37. She's a successful graphic designer who started her own business five years ago. She had no idea how stressful running a business would be, especially with a family to take care of and an elderly father in a nearby assisted living facility. Janie and her husband, Dave, are debating whether they should have another baby. Her biological clock is screaming "tick, tock!" But with her full plate and the stress she is under, she's not sure how she'd manage.

And some other things are happening, too. Something in her body is a little bit off and she can't put her finger on it. Janie has changed nothing about how she eats or exercises, but the needle on the scale keeps creeping upward. Her periods look like a crime scene where a horrible stabbing must have taken place. Her breasts are so tender before her period that even putting a bra on is painful. Janie is irritable and snappy with her kids. And poor Dave? He's in hiding most of the time. Her friends are talking about some of these problems, too. She wonders what's up. But what Janie doesn't realize is that while she's in the thick of living her life, her ovaries are secretly making their retirement plan.

Speaking the Language of Perimenopause

Before we get started, it's important to understand the terms and where you are in this transition. If you're in your late 30s to early 40s and you're experiencing the signs Janie experienced, chances are that you may be entering perimenopause. Perimenopause is the entire time from when you start noticing changes in your body that aren't garden-variety premenstrual syndrome (PMS) until the day of menopause. This can span a period of five to fourteen years. During this time, estrogen levels are rising and falling, progesterone is dropping like a rock, and testosterone may be increasing and then decreasing as you reach menopause (chin hairs, anyone?). All of this can add up to a lot of unpleasant symptoms. Menopause, on the other hand, is one day of your life. It is the day that marks one year since your last period. The average age at which this happens is 51, but there is a wide range of what is normal. I am 58 and still not yet "official." Everything that comes after the one-day menopause event is post-menopause.

If you scan the internet, you'll see multiple mentions of the "34 symptoms" of perimenopause and menopause. Is that the right number? I'm not sure. I've seen numbers into the 60s as well. What I do know is that hormone ups and downs can cause a lot of really odd experiences. The story in the beginning of the chapter is pretty typical, there are less common symptoms such as burning tongue, itchy skin, and electric shock feelings. Yes, these can be part of perimenopause too. A friend asked me why I started the book with all the symptoms and possible misery when my focus is on making perimenopause a positive experience. My focus is on the positive, but the women I meet are generally not there yet. They are scared and wondering if something is seriously wrong. With that said, here's a rundown of the most common symptoms. If you see yourself in this list, chances are that nothing is seriously wrong. You probably have a hormone imbalance, and knowing that, you can take steps to make perimenopause the positive experience it can be.

"I'm so tired!"

Fatigue is one of the most common perimenopause symptoms. It is an ongoing and persistent feeling of weakness, tiredness, and lowered energy levels, rather than just sleepiness or drowsiness. Fatigue in perimenopause can have several origins. The first is a drop in estrogen. Estrogen regulates energy at a cellular level, so when hormone levels drop during perimenopause, so do energy levels.

The second major contributor to fatigue in perimenopause is cortisol dysregulation; specifically, low cortisol, which is the stress hormone. This drop happens when you don't manage your unrelenting stress. Your body is not able to produce cortisol in quantities that match the level of stress, and the resulting fatigue screams "rest!"

The third cause of fatigue is hypothyroidism. Hormone testing can help identify which of these imbalances is causing the fatigue problem. I work with clients to interpret their hormone testing results and recommend a personalized approach to hormone balancing. You can learn more at: www.drannagarrett.com/test-and-talk.

"Where's my hair?"

Hair loss, one of the most outwardly noticeable and distressing perimenopause symptoms, is caused by estrogen deficiency because hair follicles need estrogen to sustain hair growth. Hair loss may be sudden or gradual, or manifest as thinning hair on the head or other parts of the body, including the pubic area. Hair may also become drier and more brittle, and may fall out more while brushing or in the shower.

Gradual hair loss or thinning of hair without any accompanying symptoms is common; however, for many women this symptom is upsetting, as it is a visible sign of aging. Other reasons for hair loss that should be considered in addition to low estrogen include low thyroid, high testosterone, and low iron.

"I can't concentrate."

Many perimenopausal women are concerned to find they experience mental blocks or have difficulty concentrating. This can be confusing or worrying for women, and it can have a big impact on all aspects of daily life. The main reason these symptoms occur during perimenopause is estrogen deficiency. However, not getting enough sleep can also contribute to memory problems and cause difficulty concentrating.

"Wait, why did I come into this room?"

Women in perimenopause often complain of memory loss or lapses. Misplaced car keys, skipped appointments, forgotten birthdays, and fumbling for words might seem like trivial occurrences, but these can be extremely distressing for women who have never missed a beat before. However, these memory lapses are common in perimenopause and are usually related to low levels of estrogen and/or high stress levels.

"I'm feeling dizzy"

Dizziness is a symptom of many medical conditions; however, it is also associated with perimenopause, and is caused by fluctuations in hormonal levels. Women who experience unexplained dizzy spells should consult their doctor to rule out more serious causes.

"Gotta go, gotta go right now!"

Incontinence (politely called Light Bladder Leakage or LBL) is related to falling estrogen levels. However, it can also be caused by weak pelvic floor muscles. There are three types of incontinence. Stress incontinence is the accidental release of urine while laughing, coughing, sneezing, or due to overexertion. This usually happens when the internal muscles fail to work effectively because of age, surgery, or childbirth. With urge incontinence, the bladder develops a mind of its own, contracting and emptying whenever full, despite your conscious efforts to resist. The third type is called overflow incontinence is caused by the absence of the sensation of a full bladder. This results in accidental urination because you don't realize the bladder is full.

Before you buy pads to solve the problem, try working with a pelvic physiotherapist to strengthen muscles or try bladder training exercises. It's also helpful to avoid foods that are bladder irritants, such as caffeine and spicy foods.

"I look like I'm seven months pregnant!"

Abdominal bloating is characterized by a swollen belly, a feeling of tightness, and discomfort or pain in the stomach area. Typically, it results from intestinal gas caused by low levels of bile along with estrogen deficiency. Other causes of bloating include food intolerances or leaky gut. Persistent, unexplained bloating or stomach pain for more than three days should be checked by a doctor as it can be a symptom of something more serious.

"I suddenly have hay fever."

Hormones and the immune system are intimately linked, so hormonal changes during perimenopause can lead to an increase in allergies among menopausal women. Many women experience increased sensitivity to allergens or smells, while others may suddenly become allergic to something that never bothered them before. This is particularly the case with hay fever, asthma, and dermatitis. Perimenopausal women may also develop new cases of asthma.

"My nails keep breaking."

Nail appearance can tell me a lot about a person's general health and habits. There are a variety of nail changes that occur during perimenopause that could indicate an underlying problem, but the most common is brittle nails, nails that are softer, or that crack, split, or break horizontally across the top of the nail. This can indicate a nutritional deficiency (B vitamins), hormone imbalance, or thyroid problems.

"Jeez, I stink!"

Changes in body odor can make women very self-conscious. Hormonal changes cause an increase in sweat production, in response to physical symptoms such as hot flashes and night sweats, or psychological symptoms such as anxiety and panic disorder. This increase in sweat production can lead to increased body odor, even while maintaining a good personal hygiene regimen. Increased stinkiness may also be due to genetic predisposition.

The most effective way to reduce body odor is to reduce the level of stress you are experiencing since "stress sweat" is the smelliest kind. Other ways to manage include balancing hormones, wearing lighter fabrics, or trying a chlorophyllin supplement that can help neutralize odor-causing compounds in the body.

"My heart is pounding!"

One cause of skipped beats or rapid, pounding heart-beat may be the rising FSH (follicle-stimulating hormone) that accompanies perimenopause, as the body tries harder to stimulate ovulation. The estrogen dominance and progesterone deficiency common in perimenopause adds to this scenario. For some women, heart palpitations are early signs of perimenopause and progesterone deficiency.

As with any heart condition, this symptom could signify something more serious, so it's important to report it to your healthcare provider. Stress, anxiety, and panic disorder are all other causes of this symptom that should be explored before considering a treatment option. Other triggers of irregular heartbeat to be avoided include alcohol, caffeine, and nicotine.

"I have a headache...again."

Headaches can be caused by a variety of factors such as muscle tension or drinking too much alcohol, or as a side effect of common illnesses such as the flu. However, headaches are also linked with the effects of hormonal imbalance, and therefore with the various stages of reproductive life.

Many women with regular menstrual cycles get headaches or migraines just before their periods or at ovulation. These headaches, sometimes called "menstrual migraines," occur when estrogen levels plunge during the menstrual cycle. So, as the body begins slowing down its production of estrogen during perimenopause, women may experience more frequent and intense headaches. Severe headaches that are accompanied by confusion or high fever can indicate a serious health condition and require the immediate attention of a doctor.

"My joints hurt."

Joint pain is one of the most common symptoms of perimenopause and menopause. More than half of all perimenopausal women experience varying degrees of joint pain. Estrogen helps prevent inflammation in the joints, so falling levels of estrogen during perimenopause can lead to increased inflammation, and therefore increased joint pain. Lifestyle changes are the first step to manage joint pain. I have had clients who completely cleared up their pain by eliminating sugar and gluten. Why? These foods can be very inflammatory for many women. Other inflammatory foods include corn, eggs, dairy, and soy. An elimination diet can help identify the culprits. Eliminate all of these foods for at least two weeks to see if joint pain improves, then add them back (one every three days) to see if joint pain worsens.

"My mouth is on fire."

One of the strangest symptoms of perimenopause is burning tongue or mouth. Burning mouth syndrome is a complex condition in which a burning pain occurs on the tongue or lips, or throughout the whole mouth, without visible signs of irritation, but accompanied with other symptoms such as bad breath or a bad taste in the mouth. Burning tongue affects women seven times more than men.

Low estrogen levels are thought to damage bitter taste buds in the mouth, setting off the surrounding pain neurons. Women who have persistent pain or soreness in their tongue, lips, gums, or other areas of their mouth should seek the advice of their doctor.

Gum problems are also common among perimenopausal women. The most common of the gum problems experienced in perimenopause is gingivitis, or inflammation and bleeding of the gums. Left untreated, gum problems can lead to tooth loss, infections, and heart disease, so it is important to seek treatment. Bleeding and sore gums are easy to reverse if they are caught early, with a combination of dental hygiene and tackling the underlying hormonal imbalance. If the problem continues, seek advice from a doctor or dentist.

"I just felt a shock!"

This symptom presents as a weird, "electric" sensation, like the feeling of a rubber band snapping between skin and muscle. Alternatively, when it appears as a precursor to a hot flash, it is often felt across the head. Electric shocks usually only occur for a brief moment, but it can still be quite unpleasant. The cause of electric shock sensation in perimenopause is thought to be related to the effect of fluctuating estrogen levels on the cardiovascular and nervous systems. Although this symptom is relatively harmless, it can be uncomfortable, and can be resolved by treating the underlying hormone imbalance.

"Ugh, my stomach is a mess."

Many women experience changes in gastrointestinal function, with symptoms such as excessive gas production, gastrointestinal cramping, acid reflux, and nausea. There are a couple of reasons why perimenopausal women might experience more digestive problems. First, hormone imbalance disrupts the natural transit of food in the gut. It takes longer for food to move through, and bacteria have more of an opportunity to ferment the food and create gas. Second, stress has an adverse effect on the normal functioning of hormones and can result in gut problems. Probiotics and digestive enzymes can provide support for healthy gut functioning; also, make sure you chew food well, since the digestive process starts in the mouth and doing so will decrease the amount of work your stomach and intestines need to do.

"I'm so itchy."

When estrogen levels drop during perimenopause, collagen production also slows down. Collagen is responsible for keeping skin toned, fresh-looking, and resilient. So when the body starts running low on collagen, it shows up in the skin as thinning, dryness, and a less youthful-looking appearance. To overcome itchy skin symptoms, a woman will first need to address her hormonal imbalance. Excellent hydration, sleep, and nutrition are also very important.

"What is crawling on me?"

Many women experience the feeling of 'creepy-crawlies' on their skin, a burning sensation such as an insect sting, or super-sensitivity in their hands, arms, legs, and feet. In most people, tingling is harmless, usually occurring due to a pinched nerve or compressed artery, which reduces blood flow through the extremity causing it to "fall asleep." However, in perimenopausal women, tingling extremities may be due to lower estrogen levels or a deficiency in B vitamins. Tingling extremities can also be related to anxiety, poor blood circulation, diabetes, heart disease, stroke, or a tumor. Any unexplained tingling that affects one side of the body or is accompanied by muscle weakness warrants immediate medical attention.

"I'm worried about breaking a bone."

Osteoporosis is a degenerative bone disorder, characterized by thinning and weakening of the bone and a general decrease in bone mass and density. Osteopenia is the beginning stages of osteoporosis. Thinning of bones is diagnosed by a bone density scan. Small-boned Caucasian women are at highest risk. Risk also increases if you smoke or take corticosteroid medications.

Estrogen is involved in the process of calcium absorption into the bones, so a drop in this hormone will result in an accelerated reduction in bone density from perimenopause onwards. This causes bones to be much more susceptible to breaks and fractures. The best way to improve bone density is with weight-bearing exercise. This can include walking, running, dancing or weight training. I personally reversed osteopenia by lifting heavy weights. Calcium supplementation along with Vitamin D and Vitamin K2 can also help, although calcium supplementation is controversial because of studies that have suggested that high levels of blood calcium may result in calcium deposits in arteries. Vitamin K2, which acts like a "traffic cop," keeps calcium directed toward bone building instead of being deposited in arteries.

Is it PMS or Perimenopause?

How can you tell if your symptoms are a byproduct of PMS or if they're actually signs of perimenopause? Track the frequency of your mood swings, food cravings, and other related symptoms. If they happen in the two weeks before your period and then go away, it's probably PMS. But if you're experiencing the symptoms all the time and they don't go away when your period starts, it's likely that they are related to perimenopause.

How Perimenopause Begins

Hormones begin shifting naturally around the age of 35 when estrogen and progesterone start to gradually taper off prior to menopause. In a healthy, balanced scenario, women may hardly notice this change happening in their bodies. However, for the majority of us, these hormonal shifts may overwhelm our bodies' ability to maintain balance. The result is severe symptoms that can go on for years.

The first hormone level to fall is progesterone. When perimenopause begins, you ovulate irregularly. The process of ovulation includes creation of the corpus luteum, a ripened egg that makes its way to the uterus for possible fertilization. The corpus luteum manufactures progesterone, which helps maintain pregnancy if the egg is fertilized.

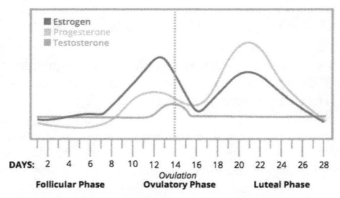

Figure 2. Hormone production pattern in a 28-day cycle

In a normal menstrual cycle (Figure 1), estrogen begins to rise markedly through the first 14 days of the cycle. After ovulation, progesterone rises to help prepare the uterus for a potential pregnancy. The progesterone has a calming, relaxing effect and helps balance estrogen. If ovulation does not occur, then no corpus luteum is produced and thus, no rise in progesterone during the luteal phase. In perimenopause, there are more cycles in which we don't ovulate, so the progesterone level stays low. This allows estrogen to run the reproductive show all month long and results in insomnia, weight gain, mood swings, breast tenderness, and changes in periods.

Understanding the Hormone Shifts of Perimenopause

An imbalance of just one hormone can throw off the rest of the symphony. That's because all hormones are made from cholesterol and are very intricately interconnected. Figure 1 shows how intimately they are related. Two important things to understand here are that pregnenolone is the "mother" hormone from which all others are created, and the body will make cortisol at the expense of all other sex hormones. Under chronic stress, pregnenolone is shuttled straight to cortisol, leaving none available to travel into the sex hormone pathway that begins with DHEA (dehydroepiandrosterone). This wreaks all kinds of havoc on hormone balance.

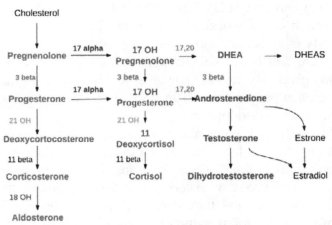

Figure 1. The hormone synthesis pathways

How can I know for sure if I'm in perimenopause?

The short answer is…you can't. Hormones are changing constantly on any given day, and a lab test only gives a snapshot of what's going on at the time of the test, so results can vary depending on that timing. Urine, blood, and saliva tests can be used to show the magnitude of the imbalance between estrogen and progesterone. Urine and saliva testing can also be used to take a look at cortisol throughout the day to see how the body is handling stress. While some physicians dismiss testing as useless because of the variability, I find it helpful for looking at the overall picture of hormone balance. All of these tests should be done between days 19 to 21 of the menstrual cycle (assuming a 28-day cycle). If you do have blood tests, your doctor will most likely test your follicle-stimulating hormone (FSH) and luteinizing hormone (LH). The higher these are, the harder your body is working to ovulate. The closer your FSH is to 50, the closer you are to menopause. Be aware that both of these test results can change on any given day, and neither gives any indication of the estrogen/progesterone balance that is the root cause of estrogen dominance.

We'll talk more about testing later in the book. Many women have met with a dismissive "Your lab tests are normal" when they are, in fact, in perimenopause. Savvy Sisters know their bodies better than anyone, and they don't settle for a brush-off from the doctor if symptoms are telling a different story.

There are things you can do that will help your symptoms

By now, you may be breaking out in a cold sweat from the fear of what is to come, but rest assured that there is plenty you can do to alleviate your symptoms. Once you're fairly sure your symptoms are related to perimenopause and a hormone imbalance, it's time to take action. The sooner you get on top of your symptoms, the easier the transition will be. Hoping it will all go away is not a good strategy because as I mentioned, perimenopause can last for five to ten years on average—or longer. That's a long time to suffer needlessly.

Lifestyle changes are foundational to having a perimenopause experience that is as benign as possible. I can't say enough about this, and I'll get into specifics in a later chapter. Here's one example of how powerful a simple change can be. I had a client who was suffering from soaking night sweats and hot flashes that would wake her up nightly. She also enjoyed two or three glasses of wine every evening to take the edge off her stress and help her get to sleep. What she didn't know was that alcohol is a major contributor to night sweats. I asked her to try skipping a few nights of wine per week to see what would happen. She did so, and her night sweats and hot flashes completely resolved on the days she skipped the wine. This was enough of a motivator for her to give up alcohol completely.

There are many powerful choices you can make to support your body. There are supplements and essential oils that can smooth the ride. But it takes WORK. There is no magic bullet. It's helpful to work with someone like me who is knowledgeable about hormone testing, interpreting test results. and options for hormone management. Many physicians are not familiar with the intricacies of hormone imbalance and, truthfully, don't have the time to get into the details of your personal puzzle. Consider looking outside the traditional medical box. Your pharmacist, an herbalist, a functional medicine doctor, or a naturopath can be an excellent resource for help.

Chapter 2:
What's Up with the
Weight Gain?

Jennifer opens her eyes, stretches in bed, and wonders what news the scale will have for her this morning. She pads slowly toward the bathroom, feeling guilty about the dessert she ate last night. She pees, then off comes her robe. Jennifer holds her breath and steps up. Her heart sinks. She's gained 0.3 pounds since yesterday and quickly decides she'll weigh again after she's had a bowel movement and make that number her "official" weight for the day. She looks in the mirror with disgust. Where did that spare tire around her middle come from? When did she start to look so old? Jennifer lets out a heavy sigh and heads for the kitchen.

She feels her stomach rumbling but decides to ignore it and grabs a cup of coffee. Breakfast is definitely out of the question since she gained. She sits down with her food tracker and reviews yesterday's entries. She's tired of thinking about every single bite she puts in her mouth, but she is sure that if she stops keeping track, she'll completely go off the rails. Dessert last night added 300 calories to her usual 1,200 for the day. She'll definitely need to work THAT off today. Jennifer dresses for the gym and heads out to her exercise class. When she first started Crossfit, the workouts energized her and made her feel strong and powerful. But now, they mostly leave her drained and exhausted the rest of the day. She decides to add in an extra run at the end of the day to make up for last night's dessert...yes, that should do it.

She's super busy at work today and only has time to grab something from the vending machine. Not too many healthy options in there. A5...out comes the package of almonds. Then she moves on to the soda machine for a Diet Coke. By mid-afternoon, she lays her head on her desk and feels like weeping because she's so tired. The waistband of her pants is digging into her middle and it's really uncomfortable, but she doesn't want to buy a larger size because that will be admitting defeat. She spends the next five minutes berating herself because she can't lose weight. Jennifer feels like a complete failure and has no idea what to do. And her frustration is starting to spill into other parts of her life.

Last night, she and her partner had a great evening out to celebrate her partner's raise. When they got home, her partner took her in his arms and suggested that they make love. Her stomach sank, and she made some lame excuse about an early meeting. But the truth is that she's very uncomfortable with him seeing her naked body. These rejections are happening more and more and it's starting to erode the edges of their relationship.

Jennifer visited her doctor to discuss these issues two weeks ago. His advice was "Eat less and move more." And he offered to write her a prescription for an appetite suppressant, which she politely declined. There was no mention of anything else that might be happening. Jennifer had read that hormone imbalances and stress can cause weight gain, but her doctor assured her that she is too young to have hormone issues. Jennifer is totally confused, defeated and ready to throw her hands up in despair.

The Link Between Hormones and Weight Loss

One of the most common complaints I hear from clients is that they can't lose weight no matter how much they diet and exercise. This is incredibly frustrating. The thing is, it may not have anything to do with what you're doing or not doing. It may be your hormones.

All hormonal imbalances can make weight loss feel difficult, if not impossible. Unfortunately, the most common issues can't be solved by dieting alone or by exercising until you drop. In fact, dieting and exercise can actually promote weight gain in some situations. If you haven't been successful with weight loss during perimenopause, chances are, one or more the following hormonal imbalances could be the problem.

High insulin and insulin resistance

Poor regulation of insulin is at the root of unwanted weight gain. Insulin is a peptide hormone that's made in the pancreas, an organ containing clusters of cells called islets. Beta cells within the islets make insulin and release it into the blood. Insulin maintains normal blood sugar levels by helping cells take in glucose; regulating carbohydrate, lipid, and protein metabolism; and promoting cell division and growth. It plays a major role in regulating how the body uses digested food for energy. With the help of insulin, glucose is absorbed by the body's cells and used for energy. Insulin's main function is to process carbohydrates in the bloodstream and carry it into cells to be used as fuel or stored as fat.

The main reasons for extra insulin include stress, eating too many nutrient-poor carbohydrates (the type found in processed foods, sugary drinks and sodas, packaged low-fat foods, and artificial sweeteners), low protein and fat intake, and low fiber consumption.

Heart palpitations, sweating, poor concentration, weakness, anxiety, fogginess, fatigue, irritability, and impaired thinking are common short-term side effects of high insulin. Our bodies typically respond to these unpleasant feelings by making us think we're hungry, which causes us to head for the vending machine or kitchen to grab high-sugar foods and drinks. It's a vicious cycle that furthers weight gain and increases the risk of diabetes and heart disease.

If insulin levels are chronically high, insulin resistance may develop. In this situation, the cells become insensitive to insulin and refuse to "open the door" to let glucose in. The pancreas senses high blood glucose because it's not going into the cells and cranks out more insulin to try to take care of the problem. Ultimately, the pancreas gets tired and stops responding to elevated blood sugar with more insulin. The end result of this insulin resistance is type 2 diabetes. You are at highest risk for developing insulin resistance if you have a family history of type 2 diabetes, or if you've had gestational diabetes, high blood pressure, or are overweight. "Apple-shaped" women who carry their fat around the middle of their bodies are more prone to insulin resistance, as are women with abnormal cholesterol. And the "apples" are at higher risk of heart disease, which is the number one killer of menopausal women. If you believe you are at risk, talk with your healthcare provider. Your blood sugar and insulin levels can be tested to give you and your doctor more information.

Imbalanced estrogen/progesterone ratio

Researchers have identified excess estrogen to be as great a risk factor for obesity as poor eating habits and lack of exercise. There are two ways to accumulate excess estrogen in the body: we either produce too much of it on our own, or we are exposed to it in our environment or diet. We're constantly exposed to estrogen-like compounds in foods that contain toxic pesticides, herbicides, and growth hormones. These molecules bind to the estrogen receptors, which allows more free, unbound estrogen to circulate. We are living in an environmental sea of estrogen imitators, and researchers are only beginning to identify the extent of this exposure on the health of humans and other species.

To compound all of this even further, fat cells make estrogen, so the more fat tissue you have, the higher your estrogen is likely to be. There are a number of ways to get the ratio of estrogen to progesterone in better balance so that weight loss is easier.

Avoid exposure to fake estrogens (xenoestrogens)

Xenoestrogens are compounds that are structurally similar to estrogen. They attach to the estrogen receptor and block the real estrogen from doing its job. These impostors are found in cosmetics, sunscreens, pesticides, plastic wrap, plastic shoes, and plastic containers (among other things). Unless you live in a bubble, it is difficult to completely avoid all of these things.

There are some simple steps you can take to cut down on your exposure. These include microwaving food in glass containers instead of plastic, using natural cleaning products, using sunscreens with physical barriers such as titanium and zinc oxide, and taking care to make sure your cosmetics are free of xenoestrogens. Anything applied to your skin will be absorbed into the body. The Environmental Working Group website (www.ewg.org) has a comprehensive list of compounds that have estrogenic properties.

Increase dietary fiber

Estrogen is metabolized in the liver, then eliminated through bowel movements. Any issues with constipation allow recirculation of the metabolites, thus worsening estrogen dominance. Fiber helps move things along in your gastrointestinal tract, which keeps estrogen moving out of the body. Most Americans eat about 20 grams per day. Aim for 35–40 grams of fiber per day but increase gradually. A sudden increase will make your GI tract very unhappy. High-fiber foods include raspberries, black beans, lentils, avocados, lima beans, split peas, and bran flakes. Flax seed is also high in fiber, but it has estrogenic properties so may worsen perimenopause symptoms in some women.

Avoid alcohol

I know. This is a total buzz-kill. But if you're serious about losing weight, you need to know that alcohol increases estrogen levels and decreases progesterone levels. It's associated with headaches, mood problems, and premenstrual anxiety, as well as an increased risk of breast cancer if you consume more than three to six servings per week. So if you're struggling with estrogen dominance, try eliminating alcohol to assess whether or not it makes a difference. Alcohol also increases belly fat. It's burned preferentially as a fuel source by your body because it is so refined, so once your body has met its caloric requirements from alcohol, the energy from any food you eat gets stored as fat.

Control stress

Chronic stress can deplete progesterone because it is diverted into the production of cortisol (which your body requires above all other hormones). This depletion will make symptoms of estrogen dominance worse. Unfortunately, we live in a world where chronic stress is the norm. But as far as your body is concerned, it is *not* normal. If you are under large amounts of stress and you're experiencing a lot of symptoms along with weight gain, your body is speaking to you. Juggling work, kids, and perhaps elderly parents can take a toll on the most even-keeled woman. Perimenopause is a perfect time to look at your commitments under a microscope and weed out any that don't truly align with your "absolute yesses." The "disease to please" will kill you by degrees (literally) because chronically high cortisol contributes to total body breakdown.

Consider supplements to balance progesterone and estrogen

There are two ways to balance estrogen and progesterone. You can either lower estrogen or increase progesterone. There are a number of supplements and essential oils that can help with this. When it comes to increasing progesterone, the first supplement I recommend is Vitamin C. In women with luteal phase defect (meaning that you don't produce enough progesterone in the second half of your cycle), Vitamin C has been shown to increase progesterone levels by about 50 percent. Herbs such as chasteberry (vitex agnus-castus) are especially helpful for newly perimenopausal women. Chasteberry has been used for more than 2,000 years and is well-researched in at least five randomized clinical trials. The way it works is unclear, but the thinking is that it increases the level of luteinizing hormone from the pituitary gland, thus increasing progesterone levels. Chasteberry works best in women who are early in the perimenopause process.

DIM (diindolylmethane) is the primary break-down product of indole 3-carbinol (I3C), a phyto-chemical found in cruciferous vegetables such as cabbage, cauliflower, broccoli, Brussels sprouts, kale, collards, mustard greens, radishes, watercress, and turnips. DIM has been shown to reduce the risk of breast, cervical and other estrogen-driven cancers cancer by helping the body create a better balance of the "good" estrogen metabolites compared to the riskier "bad" metabolite (4-hydroxyestrone) as estrogen is metabolized in the liver. DIM can also lower overall estrogen levels, so it's important to know where your estrogen/progesterone balance is before taking this. Otherwise, you may end up creating low estrogen symptoms such as hot flashes and night sweats. Possible side effects of DIM include nausea, diarrhea, and change in urine color (pink-orange). This supplement should not be used by pregnant or nursing women.

Supplementing progesterone with a bioidentical cream or capsules is another option for improving the balance between estrogen and progesterone. This is a good option for women who are nearing menopause or are already there. Bioidentical progesterone is the same compound your body makes in the ovaries. It is made from a compound called diosgenin, which is found in wild yams, but it must be chemically altered in a lab to become bioidentical progesterone. It is not the same as wild yam cream. Progesterone cream elevates body temperature slightly and for this reason, it may help with weight loss (in addition to balancing the effects of high estrogen). Oral progesterone capsules are another option. These are most useful for women who don't like applying creams or need help for perimenopausal insomnia.

Thyme essential oil has progesterone-balancing effects. It works by improving progesterone production. When used alone or with other oils such as clary sage and geranium, using thyme oil is a great way to naturally balance hormones. It is also helpful for relieving mood swings, hot flashes, and problems with insomnia. Essential oils should be used with care. They should be diluted with a carrier oil such as almond, avocado, or unfractionated coconut before being applied to the skin. Don't take them internally without the advice of an expert.

The Cortisol Connection to Weight Gain

Cortisol can be your best friend or your worst enemy. If a speeding train is heading toward you, cortisol is your BFF for sure…a rush of it will spur you to jump out of the way. But in overdoses, it's the "mean girl" in your body's neighborhood. Cortisol is one of your body's stress hormones, and it is released in stressful situations. Your body must have cortisol to live, and so production of this hormone occurs at the expense of all others. On a short-term basis, this is healthy. Long-term, however, it can lead to sex hormone imbalances, chronic illness, body breakdown, weight gain around the waist, and adrenal fatigue. Cortisol also blocks the action of thyroid hormones and progesterone, creating all kinds of hormone havoc.

If all unwanted weight gain can be related back to insulin dysregulation, you may be wondering how cortisol plays into this. When your body releases a burst of cortisol, your blood sugar goes up to give you the energy you may need to fight the tiger or avoid the speeding train. If you don't use that glucose, your body has to do something with it, so insulin is released to handle it and your liver converts it to fat. As you learned earlier in the chapter, the more insulin is released, the less sensitive your body becomes to it. Chronically high cortisol means your pancreas is working overtime to produce insulin.

Unfortunately, we live hectic lives and have become numb to stress in many ways. Something can be stressful to your body without you actually feeling the stress in a big way (like winning the lottery). Other stresses are lack of sleep, eating at irregular times, and overtraining, all of which can contribute to cortisol overdoses and therefore weight gain. The following adjustments may help.

Get enough sleep

There are reams of data that prove sleeping less than six hours a night leads to weight gain. We don't need more studies. We need to go to bed. Seven to eight hours a night is ideal.

Eat on a regular schedule

Your body expects to be fed at regular intervals. When that doesn't happen, it thinks it's starving. Cortisol rushes in to save the day by preserving fat stores. This is exactly what you don't want. If you are so busy that you forget to eat, set an alarm that reminds you to do this. Include plenty of protein, fiber, and healthy fats to keep blood sugar swings to a minimum.

Be gentle on your body

When I trained for the Susan G. Komen 3-Day walk in 2011, I walked miles and miles every week. I did not lose an ounce. But after it was over, I immediately lost eight pounds. I asked my trainer what was up with that, and he said I had been overtraining (and keeping my cortisol high). When I stopped training, the weight came off. The message here is that flogging your body with more workouts isn't the answer and may backfire completely, especially if you suspect you have any degree of cortisol imbalance. Add in some yoga or a contemplative practice, or try gentle exercise like stretching or easy walking to moderate your cortisol levels.

Map your daily cortisol pattern

If you want to go deeper to determine your cortisol levels and identify adrenal issues, it's possible to map out your daily cortisol pattern to help you target your management efforts. This can be done with a simple saliva or urine test, and your results should be interpreted by an expert. Vitamins C and B5 can be helpful for normalizing cortisol. Adaptogenic herbs such as ashwagandha, rhodiola, holy basil, and eleutherococcus are very effective for adrenal support if your pattern is abnormal (either high or low). DHEA, a hormone that is the precursor for estrogen and testosterone, is also useful for adrenal support. However, I do not recommend using DHEA without guidance. DHEA requires a prescription in some countries (e.g. Canada).

Managing weight in perimenopause starts with a foundation of good stress management: know when you can push yourself and when you need to rest. There is no magic supplement that can fix an out-of-control life, and you will never lose weight as long as your cortisol is running the show. It just can't be done. Period.

Could it be my thyroid?

When I talk with women who are experiencing unexpected weight gain, one of the first questions I am often asked is "Could it be my thyroid?" Our thyroid hormones play a huge role in regulating our metabolism and how our bodies use nutrients. As we age, the thyroid may get more sluggish, or you may develop an autoimmune thyroid problem called Hashimoto's thyroiditis. This is most common in women and results in your body attacking your thyroid gland, believing it to be "foreign."

Unexpected weight gain and difficulty losing weight may be one of the first signs that something's wrong. Other signs that may indicate a thyroid problem include brittle hair, dry skin, insomnia, and lack of energy. Research shows that even small changes in thyroid function can cause weight gain. In fact, many women who have been told their thyroid test results are "normal" may still have reduced thyroid function (subclinical hypothyroidism), which is enough to cause weight gain.

Both high and low blood sugar contribute to thyroid dysfunction. Hypothyroidism slows the rate of glucose uptake by cells, decreasing the rate of glucose absorption in the gut, slowing the clearance of insulin from the blood, and slowing the response of insulin to elevated blood sugar. When you're hypothyroid, your cells aren't very sensitive to glucose. So although you may have normal levels of glucose in your blood, you'll have the symptoms of hypoglycemia (fatigue, headache, hunger, irritability, etc.) because. your cells aren't getting the glucose they need. Your adrenals then release cortisol to increase the amount of glucose available to them, which causes a chronic stress response that further suppresses thyroid function.

What's the Best Diet to Follow in Perimenopause to Avoid Weight Gain?

This is the million-dollar question! Unfortunately, there is no one right answer for everyone. Your genetics will dictate a lot of how you respond to any diet plan, and in my experience, knowing this information can be helpful, especially if you're doing all the "right" things and not getting anywhere with weight loss. It is well worth the investment to work with a trained epigenetic coach for a precise, personalized plan. Some of the more popular diets are intermittent fasting, ketogenic, Paleo, and low glycemic index. Use caution and speak to a medical professional before you embark on any of them.

Intermittent Fasting (IF)

Intermittent Fasting is extremely popular, and some women have great success with this way of eating. There are various versions of IF, but the overarching concept is the same: eat whatever you want, but only during a specific time period. For example, the 5:2 program lets you eat normally five days of the week; the other two days you follow a modified fast by eating very little (500–600 calories). Another option, the time-restricted eating (TRE) method, involves eating only within an eight-hour period each day and fasting entirely for the remaining 14–16 hours. The potential benefits include quick fat loss, giving your digestive system a break, allowing your body to use fat stores for fuel and creating a different relationship with food.

But in my mind, the cons far outweigh the pros. Let's take a look at the downside. First, if you have a history of an eating disorder, this is definitely not your plan. Some experts believe IF to be an eating disorder with a fancy name. IF may do more harm than good for women. Studies show that alternate-day fasting can actually lower glucose tolerance and potentially wreck your metabolism. Other research shows IF can cause insomnia, anxiety, irregular periods, and hormonal imbalances. IF can also cause the following problems:

Elevated cortisol levels
Skipping meals raises your stress cortisol. Chronically high cortisol results in extra fat storage and muscle breakdown. I've known people who did IF and actu-

ally gained weight because the body thought is was in starvation mode.

An obsession with food

Hunger is a powerful evolutionary mechanism that kept us alive back in the day. Food is everywhere, so hunger isn't normally an issue we have to deal with anymore. The problem is that when you're starving, your natural tendency is to focus on eating all the time. This can create an obsession with food and spending all of your mental energy planning your next meal.

Coffee dependence

Most IF plans allow caffeine, which can keep you going for hours when you're not eating. Depending on your genetics, this may increase sleep issues and anxiety. Coffee also exacerbates your already-high cortisol levels, making fat burning more difficult and potentially breaking down muscle.

A tendency to overeat

Even if you've never done IF, you know the feeling of missing lunch and then mowing down everything in sight at dinner. We've all been there. The caloric-restriction benefit of IF disappears if your next meal becomes a free-for-all, especially if you're eating unhealthy foods.

Potentially increased food intolerances

Hunger can override any sense of logic or discipline. Several IF experts encourage a "free for all" during your eating hours so you don't feel deprived. But this can set up a food-intolerance nightmare that sets the stage for blood sugar spikes and crashes, cravings, leaky gut, and increased inflammation, depending on the food choices you make.

Ketogenic Diet

The ketogenic (keto) diet has been around for more than nine decades. It was originally created to help manage seizures in epileptic patients. It is a very low-carbohydrate (<20 gm/day), high-fat diet that puts the body into ketosis. The compounds that are produced are then burned as a fuel source. The keto diet targets hormone imbalances, especially insulin resistance and high blood sugar levels. The high fat, moderate protein approach in this diet helps keep hunger under control and keeps blood sugar levels steady. This also helps keep cortisol levels steady.

The pitfalls of this plan are that it can be hard to follow (70–80 percent of calories as fat is a lot), a person's intake of unhealthy fats may increase to meet the fat requirements, and there is some evidence that suggests this plan may contribute to thyroid problems. Many women do not do well with this low level of carbohydrates and experience brain fog and low energy. Knowing your genetics can help you assess whether this plan will work for you.

Paleo Diet

The Paleo diet has been associated with many health benefits from better blood sugar levels to reduced inflammation. It's considered one of the best diet plans for weight loss because it's high in protein and fat and emphasizes whole foods. However, it's also been the subject of much controversy in recent years because of claims that it could prevent or cure certain illnesses, and the fact that it eliminates certain food groups such as grains and dairy.

The Paleo diet plan is very popular and there is a huge following of people who swear by it. The Paleo diet definition is simple: eat only foods that were available to our hunter and gatherer ancestors thousands of years ago during the Paleolithic Age. This means that things like processed foods, refined grains, and cereals are off the menu, replaced with fruits and vegetables, meats, nuts, and seeds. Because it is essentially a grain-free diet, it tends to be lower in carbohydrates and higher in protein and fat than some other diets.

Low Glycemic Index

The glycemic index is a tool that's used to indicate how a particular food affects blood sugar (or glucose) levels. The definition of the glycemic index (GI) is "a measure of the blood glucose-raising potential of the carbohydrate content of a food compared to a reference food (generally pure glucose or sugar)." Foods are assigned a glycemic index number based on how quickly they raise blood sugar compared to pure glucose. Pure glucose has a glycemic index number of 100, meaning that it's broken down rapidly by the body and increases blood sugar very quickly. Any excess glucose is saved in the muscles as glycogen for later use, or stored inside fat cells when there's a surplus.

All foods containing glucose, fructose, or sucrose (various forms of carbohydrates or sugars) can be classified as high GI, moderate GI, or low GI. The glycemic index values of all foods range from 0–100:

- High GI = 70 and above
- Moderate GI = 55 to 69
- Low GI = below 55

Whenever we eat any type of carbohydrate, whether it's pure sugar or a cup of fresh vegetables, the molecules in the food are broken down as they're absorbed. This impacts blood glucose levels and insulin release.

The speed with which a carbohydrate causes this process to happen depends on how quickly it is broken down; some carbs that are low on the glycemic index (veggies and 100 percent whole grains, for example) cause a smaller and more gradual rise in blood glucose, while carbs that have a high glycemic (soda and white potatoes) cause rapid glucose absorption and high insulin release. Low GI carb choices include brown or wild rice, sweet potatoes, sprouted ancient grains, legumes, and beans, while poor choices include sugary drinks, white rice, and white bread Choosing low glycemic foods helps keep insulin levels steady, thus helping with weight gain and chronic health problems such as type 2 diabetes or prediabetes, heart disease, hypertension, and obesity. Foods that are pure fat or protein (meat, cheese, oils and eggs) have a glycemic index of 0 because they contain no carbohydrates.

Weight gain in perimenopause can be frustrating, and there is no one right answer for addressing it. Rather than focus on one specific diet, I recommend that my clients focus on eating whole, nutrient-dense foods that are varied and colorful. Rarely do I recommend eliminating entire food groups unless there's a good reason to (such as a clear sensitivity to a particular food). Weight loss requires a multi-pronged approach to regulate insulin levels, manage stress, and solve any underlying hormone imbalances.

Chapter 3:
Is Perimenopause
Stealing Your Sleep?

Angela is barely functioning. As a freelance writer, she needs to be on top of her game to keep her clients happy and the jobs flowing in. It's the third night in a row that she's woken up every hour or two with hot flashes. She rolls out of the hot spot on the mattress, flings off the covers, flips her pillow to the cool side and takes a peek at the clock. 3:30 a.m. Ugh. She has a 7:00 a.m. meeting and wonders whether she has enough eye drops to get the red out. They'll probably think she's been drinking, which at this point doesn't sound like a bad idea. Night after night, she stares at the ceiling, wondering what is going on and when this torture will end. She's drinking more caffeine than ever. And three glasses of wine now seem to be the magic number to get her to sleep. But dear Lord, the hot flashes come all night long! Finally, at 4:00 a.m., she gets up and turns on the coffee. Time to try to survive another day.

Why do so Many Women Suffer with Insomnia in Perimenopause?

Insomnia is one of the most distressing problems that women experience in perimenopause. It's not life-threatening, but a lack of sleep affects every part of our mental and physical being. Studies show that even moderate sleep deprivation (less than 6 hours per night) results in a performance equivalent to driving drunk. Nearly nine million Americans depend on sleeping pills to get a good night's sleep. Unfortunately, sleeping pills only add about 40 minutes to the time you're asleep, and they carry a high risk for dependency.

There are many variations on the insomnia theme: waking at the same hour every night; waking multiple times during the night; racing thoughts; heart palpitations; night sweats; and hot flashes. Occasionally, a client of mine will have difficulty falling asleep, but most complain of broken sleep in the wee hours of the morning. Although the causes may differ, the result is the same. All of them drag through their days and feel as if they can barely function.

The relationship between sleep and hormones is complex and often confusing. Part of the reason is that there are so many different hormones carrying messages through your body while still connected to one another. That means if one is not at an optimal level, it may skew others, and several are impacted by how much sleep you get. At the same time, hormone levels (particularly those that are too high or too low) can directly affect your ability to get to sleep or stay asleep.

Low progesterone and high cortisol wreak havoc on sleep

Low levels of progesterone (the most common hormone imbalance in perimenopause) contribute to sleep problems. In perimenopause, lack of ovulation leads to dramatic drops in progesterone. When low progesterone is your problem, you'll most likely be waking up at 1:00 or 2:00 a.m. In addition to an imbalance of sex hormones during perimenopause, a lot of women suffer from high levels of cortisol, which can contribute significantly to chronic insomnia.

In a perfect world, your cortisol levels are high in the morning and gradually decrease during the day to very low levels at bedtime. But in our overstressed world, many women have a bedtime rise in cortisol. This interferes with restorative REM sleep and interrupts sleep rhythms. That's why so many women in perimenopause say they are able to fall asleep, but they can't stay asleep. High cortisol levels can also cause racing, panicky thoughts, heart palpitations, and even panic attacks. If you have high levels of cortisol, you will not be able to sleep even if you are exhausted and you may find yourself waking at 4:00 a.m. when cortisol normally rises.

I am a sleep fanatic. So much so that at my annual New Year's Eve party, I have *one* rule. Everyone must be gone by 10:00 p.m. My friends know this and are actually appreciative that they can go home and get a good night's sleep, too. Insomnia has been my personal piece of perimenopause hell and it has taken me a long time to stumble on the magic formula that helps. Part of the solution was finding a mouthpiece to keep my husband from snoring…but I digress. (I'll share my personal "sleep-stack" at the end of this chapter.)

We all know that lack of sleep makes you cranky and bitchy. But you may not be familiar with all the other, less well-known reasons you need to be sleeping seven to eight hours a night. Let's take a look.

Lack of sleep makes you dumb
Sleep plays a critical role in thinking and learning. Lack of sleep interrupts these processes. First, it impairs attention, alertness, concentration, reasoning, and problem solving. This makes it more difficult to learn efficiently. Second, during the night, various sleep cycles play a role in "consolidating" memories in the mind. If you don't get enough sleep, you won't be able to remember what you learned and experienced during the day. I don't know about you, but I need all the help I can get in this department!

Your sex drive goes down the drain
Sleep-deprived men and women report lower libidos and less interest in sex. Depleted energy, sleepiness, and amped-up crankiness may be largely to blame.

It's depressing
Lack of sleep and sleep disorders can contribute to the symptoms of depression. In one survey, people who were diagnosed with depression or anxiety were more likely to sleep less than six hours per night. Insomnia is often one of the first symptoms of depression. It's a vicious cycle because lack of sleep aggra-

vates the symptoms of depression, and depression can make it more difficult to fall asleep.

It makes you look old
Most people have experienced eye bags after a few nights of missed sleep. But chronic sleep loss can lead to dull skin, fine lines, and dark circles under the eyes. Cortisol is a player when it comes to skin too. High cortisol can break down skin collagen, the protein that keeps skin smooth and elastic.

It can kill you before your time
British researchers looked at how sleep patterns affected the mortality of more than 10,000 British civil servants over two decades. The results, published in 2007, showed that those who cut their sleep from seven to five or fewer hours a night nearly doubled their risk of death from all causes. In particular, lack of sleep doubled the risk of death from cardiovascular disease.

Your judgment suffers (especially when it comes to sleep)
Lack of sleep can affect our ability to interpret events. This hurts our decision-making if we are not accurately assessing a particular situation. Sleep-deprived people seem to be especially prone to poor judgment when it comes to assessing what lack of sleep is doing to them. In our society, functioning on no sleep has become a kind of badge of honor. You may think you're doing fine, but the odds are high that you're wrong. And if you work in a profession where it's important to be able to judge your level of functioning, this can be a big problem.

Strategies to Manage Sleep Problems in Perimenopause

When I'm working with clients (especially those who suspect they may have adrenal issues), sleep is the first place we start when it comes to lifestyle changes. This is the number one thing you can change that will quickly make a big difference in your mental and physical health.

You now know there are two central problems that cause insomnia in perimenopause: low progesterone and high cortisol. Each of these has different management strategies, but first, let's focus on lifestyle changes that can be helpful for insomnia. The most obvious way to control cortisol is to reduce stress. That, however, is easier said than done for most of us. But while you can't just press an "off" button on your life, there are changes that can help. Consider these ideas to calm your brain and increase the likelihood of sleep:

- Learn to say "no." And yes, that's a complete sentence.
- Sometimes "good enough" is good enough. Be willing to accept imperfection.
- Get regular exercise, but not too close to bedtime.
- Shut down screens at least an hour before bedtime. Blue light interferes with melatonin production.
- Try a magnesium supplement before bed. Magnesium is a calming mineral. I like magnesium glycinate because it's the least likely

of the magnesium supplements to cause diarrhea.

Can't I just fix this with wine?

Let's be honest. Wine is a perimenopausal go-to for many women. It takes the edge off anxiety, overwhelm, and much of the hormonal chaos we experience. And while it can help you get to sleep faster, there are hidden dangers in this management strategy. Women metabolize alcohol differently than men. We have less water in our bodies to dilute the alcohol; fewer enzymes to digest the alcohol; smaller body size; and hormonal differences that may affect absorption. Plus, as we age, we metabolize alcohol less efficiently so blood alcohol levels stay higher longer.

According to some studies, a drink a day can actually be heart protective, but more than that can result in long-term health problems such as breast cancer. Here are more reasons to avoid this strategy:

Alcohol makes you fat
At 100 or more calories per glass of wine, it's easy to run up the calorie scoreboard. Do the math. Take the number of drinks you have per day and multiply by 365. Take that number and multiply by 100. Then divide by 3,500. The result is the number of pounds you could lose over a year simply by not drinking. Plus, alcohol has no nutritional value, and it raises your cortisol and estrogen levels and throws insulin out of whack, all of which contribute to further weight gain and a bigger muffin top.

Breast cancer
Alcohol increases estrogen levels, which, over a long period of time, have been shown to increase breast cancer risk. In addition, drinking also causes your body to convert more testosterone to estradiol (a type of estrogen). And remember all that fat you're storing with extra calories? It's cranking out estrogen too.

Insomnia
Even though it can help you get to sleep faster, alcohol actually contributes to insomnia in two ways. First, it increases cortisol production. Second, it disrupts sleep patterns (even though you may fall asleep more easily). This is thought to be a result of blood sugar swings that result when alcohol wears off in the middle of the night.

Osteoporosis
Alcohol can increase the risk of osteoporosis by increasing parathyroid hormone (PTH) levels. This throws off the body's calcium balance. In cases of chronic alcohol abuse, blood levels of PTH stay elevated, which puts a strain on the body's calcium reserves in bones. Alcohol also inhibits the production of enzymes found in the liver and kidneys that convert the inactive form of vitamin D to its active form. This interference with the body's vitamin D also affects calcium absorption. Keeping your bones strong is incredibly important for overall health. Hip fractures in older women are a common cause of nursing home admissions, and one in five people with a hip fracture die within a year. Thanks, but no thanks.

Hot flashes and night sweats

Many women report that alcohol is a trigger for hot flashes and/or night sweats. Alcohol causes estrogen to rise, then once the alcohol has been metabolized, your estrogen level drops and voila! Hot flash! Stabilizing estrogen levels is key to stopping hot flashes and night sweats. Hot flashes and night sweats don't happen to all women, but if they affect you, try cutting out alcohol to see if that helps. I've had clients completely banish these perimenopause symptoms with this change alone.

More cases of alcoholism start in midlife for women than at any other time of life. This is a big deal. Empty nest syndrome, loss of identity, divorce, and chronic health problems are just a few of the reasons women turn to alcohol. Numbing behaviors may help temporarily, but drinking is a poor long-term Band-Aid⟶. It wrecks lives and health if things get out of control. If you're having trouble dealing with midlife transitions, get help. There's no shame in that. Remember, we're all in this together.

Can't I just jump-start with caffeine every morning?

If you're experiencing perimenopausal symptoms and you've done any research at all, one of the recommendations you've likely seen giving up caffeine. This is not great news for many of us. Caffeine is addictive, and the warmth of that morning coffee ritual may be deeply ingrained. I feel your pain.

Caffeine (even if consumed in the morning) may be making insomnia worse. Some people (like me) are genetically wired to be slow metabolizers of caffeine, meaning that it takes longer to be eliminated from your body. We're prone to insomnia and anxiety from caffeine. If you're sleep-deprived, your morning jolt may seem like a good plan, but it's a quick-fix, and you'll pay later with the hit that your adrenal glands take. Your morning java kicks your adrenal glands into overdrive, stimulating the production of cortisol. If your adrenals are already tired, flogging them with caffeine will make recovery that much more difficult. Been there, done that.

There are two ways to give up caffeine:

Cold turkey

This is best done when you have a few days where you don't have to be on your A-game. Or around any people. Have some ibuprofen handy. You'll feel foggy and tired and most likely have a raging headache, but this method is "quick and dirty" and the payoff at the end is worth it.

Gradual taper (my preferred method)

You can begin to mix decaf coffee into your regular coffee in increasing proportions. Start with three-quarters regular and one-quarter decaf and work your way down over a period of a few weeks. You'll still get some grogginess, but it's a much less brutal way to break up with your beloved beverage than going cold turkey.

How to get better sleep

Create a bedtime routine

The first step to address trouble sleeping is making sure your hormones are balanced. Other important foundational steps are to create a relaxing nighttime routine, unplug from electronics at least an hour before bed, and create a comfortable sleep haven in your bedroom (comfy, dark, and cool). Go to bed and get up at the same time every day. Yes, even on weekends. Avoid alcohol or large meals right before bed as both interrupt sleep. Yoga nidra or guided meditation can be very helpful for getting you to sleep.

Supplements that may help with sleep

It may be tempting to resort to over-the-counter sleep aids (most contain antihistamines) or prescription sleep medications, but these don't treat the root cause of insomnia and may lead to dependency. Over time, they also work less effectively, which means you need higher and higher doses to do the job. As someone who's been there and done that, I don't recommend this approach. Instead, get to the bottom of the problem.

Before you head to the supplement aisle and start to create your own herbal cocktail, please read Chapter 9 and consider consulting with a professional about correct dosages and what core issue you're hoping to treat.

Chasteberry

If perimenopause is a relatively recent development for you, chasteberry may be a good supplement to try. It's an herb that helps increase progesterone and it can create better balance between estrogen and progesterone.

Progesterone capsules or creams

Progesterone supplements are another option. Oral progesterone capsules (prescription only) are most effective for insomnia. When taken orally, progesterone has to pass through the liver to be metabolized, and one of the metabolites that is created, allopregnanolone, causes drowsiness. Bioidentical progesterone is very safe and has never been associated with increased cancer risk. In addition to drowsiness, side effects may include dizziness, nausea, and depression. These are rare, however, and progesterone is generally well tolerated and effective.

Over-the-counter progesterone creams can also be helpful. These are widely available in health food stores and online. Most creams contain 3 percent USP progesterone that is derived from wild yams. Please note that this is not the same as wild yam cream. Wild yams contain a substance called diosgenin that your body cannot convert to progesterone on its own, so this step must be done in a lab. The resulting compound is chemically identical to the progesterone your body makes, and thus, is bioidentical. Instructions for use vary according to whether you are still cycling regularly or not, and I recommend getting the help of a professional before undertaking this on your own, especially if you suspect you have low cortisol. If this is the case, then the progesterone may get shunted directly into cortisol production and have the opposite effect (wiring you up) from what you want.

GABA

Gamma aminobutyric acid (GABA), an amino acid, is the main inhibitory neurotransmitter in your central nervous system; your body's natural "off" switch. GABA slows nerve activity in your brain, which leads to feelings of calm and relaxation.

Many anti-anxiety medications and sleeping pills, including alprazolam (Xanax) and diazepam (Valium), work by enhancing the activity of GABA in your brain at the receptors. Some natural sedative herbs, such as valerian, also work by increasing GABA.

Research has shown favorable results using GABA supplementation. In one study, an amino acid preparation containing both GABA and 5-HTP, which your body produces from the amino acid tryptophan, reduced time to fall asleep, increased the duration of sleep and improved sleep quality.

Taurine

Taurine is an amino acid that reduces cortisol levels and increases the production of GABA. Try taking 500 mg before bed. Using magnesium taurate allows you to get both magnesium and taurine with a single pill.

Hops

Hops aren't just for beer. They have a sedative effect and are found in many sleep blends. Its actual efficacy in sleep is debatable, however, and it's likely not a good choice to manage insomnia on its own. Hops may best serve as a calming supplement and can be found in herbal sleep blends along with valerian, lemon balm and passionflower.

Passionflower

Studies suggest that passionflower may be just as effective as synthetic drugs for generalized anxiety disorder (GAD). It's common to see it combined with other calming herbs such as valerian root and lemon balm, chamomile, hops, kava, and skullcap in herbal sleep blends.

Side effects of passionflower include dizziness, confusion, involuntary muscle movement and loss of coordination, and sedation. It should be avoided if you're taking blood-thinner medications and/or an older class of antidepressant medication called monoamine oxidase inhibitors (MAOIs). Because passionflower may help lower blood pressure, caution is advised when using this herb with blood pressure medications.

Valerian root

Studies show that valerian reduces the time it takes to fall asleep and improves sleep quality, so if you can't sleep, it may be just what you're looking for. Unlike many prescription sleeping pills, valerian has fewer side effects and is a lot less likely to result in morning drowsiness.

In one double-blind study conducted by the Foellinge Health Center in Sweden, the effects of valerian on poor sleep were significant. Of the study participants, 44 percent reported perfect sleep while 89 percent reported improved sleep when taking valerian root. In addition, no side effects were observed for this group. That being said, be aware that valerian root smells like dirty socks, so don't be alarmed when you open the bottle!

Lemon balm

The ancient Mediterranean people loved lemon balm in tea form and research is validating the benefits of lemon balm is as an anti-anxiety supplement. A study of brainwaves showed that lemon balm was useful in reducing anxiety. In a separate two to four-week study, taking two doses of 300 mg lemon balm extract helped reduce anxiety by up to 15 to 18 percent in 20 participants. This same study showed that lemon balm could reduce insomnia by up to 42 percent.

Adaptogenic herbs

Adaptogens increase the capacity of the body to adapt to stress and to resist disease. They don't work on a specific body organ but have a "normalizing" effect on imbalances caused by physical or emotional stress. The herb ashwagandha has been shown to increase energy and mental alertness during the day and to help you sleep better at night. It can be taken alone (400 mg) or in a blend with other adaptogens.

Magnesium

Magnesium is an essential mineral, one of seven essential macro-minerals that your body needs in large quantities. Unfortunately, the body does not produce magnesium, so it needs to come from outside sources. Magnesium deficiency is common among adults, which leads to restless sleep and waking frequently during the night. I can personally say that magnesium has made a huge difference in my sleep.

Maintaining healthy levels of this mineral often leads to deeper, more sound sleep because it helps maintain healthy levels of GABA.

Melatonin

Melatonin is a hormone that tells your body when it is time to head to bed. Melatonin levels start to rise when it is dark outside, signaling to your body that it is time to sleep. It also binds to receptors in the body and helps with relaxation. People who don't make enough melatonin at night can struggle to fall asleep. It is a popular supplement for sleep and jet lag. Long-term chronic use can result in a decrease in the body's natural ability to produce it, so it should be used short-term.

There are many factors that may cause low melatonin levels at night. Stress, smoking, exposure to too much light at night (including blue light from screens), not getting enough natural light during the day, shift work, and aging all affect melatonin production. Taking a melatonin supplement may help counter low levels and normalize your internal clock. I generally recommend starting with one milligram about 30 minutes before bedtime.

Essential oils

The essential oils of certain herbs can work wonders when it comes to de-stressing and getting to sleep. Essential oils of lavender and roman chamomile are popular for their calming properties, but less flowery options such as marjoram, cedarwood, and bergamot also offer sleep benefits. Oils can be inhaled, diffused, or used on the bottoms of your feet (dilute in a carrier oil such as almond oil or unfractionated coconut oil). Never take oils internally unless you are working with an aromatherapy specialist.

A note on prescription sleep medications

Prescription sleep medications, such as Ambien or Lunesta can be useful when used for a short period of time to re-establish sleep. Unfortunately, many people end up staying on them long-term and become dependent on them. They all have significant side effects. According to Drugs.com, Ambien (which is the most popular sleep drug these days) has common side effects that include drowsiness, headaches, nasal congestion, memory loss, muscle aches, double vision, diarrhea, swollen lymph nodes, voice changes, forgetfulness, belching, and body aches, among others. The most alarming side effect is "sleep driving" where the person is asleep, gets behind the wheel of a car and causes an accident. Sleep eating and sleepwalking have also been reported. Women take longer to metabolize Ambien than men, and thus are more likely to suffer side effects the following day.

I am a veteran of Ambien use. Insomnia has been my constant companion since the birth of my daughter 30 years ago. I used Ambien for a couple of years and then it stopped working and I'd wake up at 2:00 a.m. Finally, I thought, "This is stupid." It took me an entire year to wean myself off. I believe that part of the problem is that I was anxious about not sleeping, so the idea of getting no sleep due to rebound insomnia was terrifying. Did I mention that I'm a sleep fanatic? I did finally stop my insomnia with the help of oral progesterone and a cocktail of herbs that I am happy to share. It includes: 400 mg oral progesterone, 400 mg magnesium glycinate at bedtime, one

capsule of ACTS (an adaptogen blend), and two capsules of End Fatigue Revitalizing Sleep formula (a
blend of nervine herbs). What works for me may not
work for you, so my advice is to work with someone
who is knowledgeable about hormones, herbs, and
oils to help you create your own special sleeping regimen.

Chapter 4:
Periods and
Perimenopause: What's
Normal and What's Not?

The day had finally come. Months before, Laura had been accepted to do a TEDx talk in her city, and she'd been practicing and perfecting her speech for what felt like ages. Now, here she was, and her excitement was over the top. Except for one problem. Her period had started yesterday, and for the last few months she had experienced terrible flooding for the first three days. Her nerves were already frayed, and now this. So, armed with a super tampon and the thickest pad she could find, she stepped out on stage.

Laura was about seven minutes into her talk when she felt the trickle of blood down her leg. Fortunately, she had worn a long skirt, but she wondered how much time she had left before the bleeding became obvious. She took a deep breath, said a silent prayer, and kept going. When she finished speaking, she rushed to the bathroom only to find a horrific mess that stopped half an inch above her hemline. Laura started to cry, partly from relief that her talk was over and she hadn't been embarrassed, and partly because she was so tired of dealing with this. She had no idea what was going on with her body, but knew she needed a solution. NOW.

Changes in Your Cycle are a Clue

Some of the most common questions I'm asked in the Hormone Harmony Club are: "What is going on with my period? Is this normal? Do I need to see my doctor?" When women enter perimenopause, all kinds of period problems become fair game. They commonly experience flooding, clots, short cycles, abnormally long periods, cramping, and symptoms that are alarming and, in some cases, life-altering. While it would be nice if there was an on/off switch when it comes to periods and perimenopause, this is not usually the case. Changes in your cycle are a tip-off that perimenopause has arrived, and there is a wide range of experiences that are all "normal."

Take me, for instance. I was a 28-day girl—just like clockwork. You could set your watch by my cycle. Then, I started having periods every two weeks. Not good! Then I'd go six weeks or so with nothing. Once, I went six months period-free and hoped the off switch was permanently pressed. But no, I had another period and started my count all over again.

For most women, the average cycle length is 25 to 31 days with bleeding that lasts about five days. Irregular periods are defined as changes in this typical cycle and are characterized by abnormal bleeding and/or unusual cycle lengths. Cycle changes can begin as early as your mid-30s and the exact symptoms of irregular periods vary. Most women experience irregular periods for three to ten years before they stop completely.

Irregular Periods

For women in perimenopause, the most likely cause of irregular periods is fluctuating hormone levels. The menstrual cycle is controlled by estrogen and progesterone, both of which begin to decline in a woman's 40s and 50s. When hormone production begins to taper off, periods begin to vary both in length and volume. During perimenopause, irregular periods are common. This is rarely cause for concern. Irregular periods occur because the usual pattern in the rise and fall of estrogen and progesterone is disrupted, resulting in unpredictable fluctuations in hormones. As a result, there are a variety of different menstrual changes that may occur, all of which are "normal." Cycles may be shorter than usual, or bleeding can be days to weeks late. Periods can be heavier, or lighter, or vary a lot between each cycle.

Short cycles

Short menstrual cycles occur when there is a very low estrogen level compared with progesterone. This is because estrogen causes the uterine lining to thicken, so when the levels are low, there is less lining to shed, hence the periods become short or light. When there are fluctuations in estrogen and progesterone levels, periods may be more frequent. While irritating and annoying, this situation is not usually a cause for a doctor's visit unless periods are happening more often than every two weeks.

Flooding and/or prolonged periods

Nothing is more disconcerting than feeling as if you are a prisoner in your home every time your period starts. I work with so many women who tell me that they can't go anywhere for the first two to three days of their cycle because they know they'll be bleeding through clothing. Ugh! The second most inconvenient problem is periods that go on for weeks or months.

Flooding or prolonged periods are both caused by an excess of estrogen that stimulates the uterine lining to grow, grow, grow. If you happen to not ovulate in a particular month, then there's nothing to signal your body to have a period, and the lining keeps on growing. When you finally do have a period, it can be extremely heavy or clot-filled (or both) and long. Not only is this annoying, it can lead to anemia over time which can result in other health problems. Low levels of red blood cells and iron contribute to fatigue, poor memory, dizziness, paleness, and other problems because inadequate amounts of oxygen are transported to the cells. Anemia can become a vicious cycle because it also makes a woman more likely to bleed more heavily.

Other conditions can also contribute to heavy bleeding. Fibroid tumors can develop in the endometrial wall and prevent the normal uterine contractions that help stop menstrual blood flow each month. Fibroids are the most common physical reason for excessive bleeding. Adenomyosis, a condition caused by growth of endometrial glands into the uterine wall, is another cause of heavy bleeding. Blood does not fully drain from the uterus each month and builds up, causing the organ to swell and be unable to contract fully. Both of these conditions are associated with high levels of estrogen and low progesterone.

There are a number of ways you can improve heavy or long periods. I like a gradual approach that begins with lifestyle changes.

1. Reduce alcohol consumption
Alcohol raises estrogen levels and can disrupt liver function. I recommend fewer than four servings a week.

2. Avoid xenoestrogens
"Fake" estrogens bind to receptors and allow more free hormones to circulate, which in turn stimulates the uterine lining to grow. These substances include plastics, pesticides and some chemicals that are found in sunscreens and cosmetics.

3. Eat less conventionally raised meat and dairy
Dairy consumption is associated with higher estradiol levels, as is eating red meat. Choose organic, grass-fed versions of these products to avoid the hormones that are used in conventional farming.

4. Up your fiber intake

Fiber is very important when it comes to controlling estrogen. It keeps things moving along in the GI tract. You eliminate most of your metabolized estrogen in bowel movements, so issues with constipation worsen estrogen dominance. I recommend increasing fiber to at least 35 grams per day. The average American eats less than 20 grams per day. Increase fiber gradually until the goal is met.

5. Lose weight

Fat cells make their own estrogen, which can make the likelihood of flooding periods higher in overweight women.

The second step after lifestyle is supplements. Remember, before you go pick up supplements to try, please read Chapter 9 and consider consulting with a professional for dosage information.

Progesterone cream, oil, or capsules

Bioidentical progesterone is a hormone that balances out estrogen, thus preventing the continual growth of the uterine lining. The choice of product largely depends on other symptoms that may be going on in addition to bleeding, or it may be a personal preference. Capsules are best used when insomnia is also an issue. Oil, which is rubbed on gums or held under the tongue, is best when you want to avoid possible buildup of progesterone in fat tissue. Cream is excellent for many symptoms, and doses can be easily adjusted. Cream and oil are available over-the-counter; capsules require a prescription. I recommend working with an expert and getting hormone testing before try this approach on your own.

Vitamin C

Vitamin C (2,000-4,000 mg/day) has an anti-estrogenic effect on the uterus. A study to see the effects of this supplement on bleeding showed it was able to reduce heavy bleeding in 87 percent of women who participated. Doses this high may cause diarrhea in some women. If this happens, try reducing the dose.

DIM (diindolylmethane) or IC3 (indole-3-carbinol)

These are both created from compounds in cruciferous vegetables and help improve estrogen metabolism and lower estrogen levels, thus improving the balance of estrogen/progesterone and reducing the likelihood of extreme uterine lining overgrowth.

Shepherd's purse

Shepherd's purse is an astringent herb that constricts blood vessels, thereby reducing blood flow. When dried and infused in a tea or tincture, it is one of the best remedies for stopping hemorrhages of all kinds.

Lady's mantle

Lady's mantle is an herb that helps relieve mild aches and pains during menstruation. It is also used in a tea or tincture to stop spotting between periods and lessen heavy bleeding. It can be used with shepherd's purse.

Iron

One of the most concerning consequences of heavy bleeding is anemia, which can cause fatigue, hair loss, shortness of breath, rapid heartbeat, dizziness, and/or paleness. Left untreated, it can lead to heart problems because the heart enlarges to compensate for the lack of red blood cells needed to transport oxygen. Anemia can also lead to irregular heartbeat. Treating anemia is straightforward in most cases by solving the underlying bleeding problem and replacing iron.

There are many products available to supplement iron. My personal preference is ferrous fumarate because it is better absorbed than ferrous sulfate, and it tends to be less hard on the stomach. Iron absorption is increased when it is taken with Vitamin C. Iron tends to be constipating (which may worsen estrogen dominance) and will turn bowel movements black. It should never be taken unless you know your levels are low because it can build up in tissues and cause toxicity and even death.

The third step to help control heavy bleeding is medications. These are available only by prescription with the exception of non-steroidal anti-inflammatory drugs (NSAIDS).

NSAIDs

Over-the-counter medications such as ibuprofen and naproxen can help control heavy bleeding, but they are not a great long-term solution as they can affect blood pressure and increase the likelihood of stomach ulcers. When used short-term during your period, however, they can be very effective at slowing bleeding. Take NSAIDs daily, starting one to two days before your period, and continue regularly through your heaviest days. Use the lowest dose that gives you results. Typical doses are 250 to 500 mg two to four times a day for naproxen and 600 to 1,200 mg/day for ibuprofen. Do not take NSAIDs if you have a stomach ulcer, kidney disease or uncontrolled high blood pressure.

Tranexamic acid

Tranexamic acid is another medication that helps decrease bleeding. Tranexamic acid works by slowing the breakdown of blood clots, which helps to prevent prolonged bleeding. It belongs to a class of drugs known as antifibrinolytics. Tranexamic acid is not a hormone, does not treat other menstrual or premenstrual symptoms. does not stop your period, is not a form of birth control, and does not protect against sexually transmitted diseases.

Birth control pills

Birth control pills are another option for heavy, frequent, or prolonged periods. They contain a combination of synthetic estrogen and progestin, or progestin only. Birth control pills shut down all of the body's hormone production so that pregnancy cannot occur. The menstrual cycle is then artificially controlled by the pill. Some brands allow for a break that induces hormone withdrawal bleeding or a "period," while others are meant to be taken all the time (thus eliminating the period). Again, these products are associated with a small increase in breast cancer risk due to the synthetic progestin, and they may have side effects that are similar to the IUD. Changing brands may help with side effects if they occur, as most side effects are related to the particular combination of hormones in the pill, which varies by brand.

A note on birth control use for irregular cycles

Doctors will often prescribe birth control pills or a hormone-releasing IUD to control irregular cycles. Birth control pills shut down hormone production completely (thus applying a Band-Aid⁻⁷ over the imbalance), but they have recently been shown, along with the progestin-containing IUDs, to increase a woman's risk of breast cancer if used long-term. A recent study, which followed 1.8 million Danish women for more than a decade, showed that for every 100,000 women, hormone contraceptive use causes an additional 13 breast cancer cases a year. That is, for every 100,000 women using hormonal birth control, there are 68 cases of breast cancer annually, compared with 55 cases a year among nonusers—and the risk increases with age. These findings support the conclusions from the 2002 Women's Health Initiative study where synthetic progestins were found to increase breast cancer risk. Synthetic progestins are the common link between combined hormone contraceptives, progestin-only pills and hormone-releasing IUDs.

The Danish study also found an increased risk for women who used contraceptives involving hormones long-term. Women who stayed on hormones for 10 or more years experienced a 38 percent increase in their relative risk of developing breast cancer as compared with nonusers. The risk persisted even after hormones were stopped. There was no increased

risk for breast cancer seen in women who used hormones for less than one year.

Medroxyprogesterone acetate

Also known as Provera, medroxyprogesterone ace-
tate is a synthetic progestin that is frequently prescribed on a short-term basis for period problems. It
has problems of its own, however, the most significant of which is that the drug was implicated in the
increased risk of breast cancer as demonstrated in the
2002 Women's Health Initiative trial of hormone
replacement. But when used short-term, it is unlikely
to cause an increase in cancer risk, and it is especially effective if you have a fibroid that bleeds, and you
haven't been able to solve your problem with other
approaches. Provera for heavy periods is prescribed
at a dose of 10 mg once or twice per day for the two
weeks before your period is due. Then you give your
body a rest for two weeks and start over. Usually a
three-month cycle of two weeks on and two weeks
off will result in a significant decrease in bleeding.
Though Provera can have side effects, these are usually acceptable compared to the option of losing your
uterus due to a hysterectomy.

Intrauterine devices

Intrauterine devices (IUD) that are impregnated with
synthetic progestins are an option to reduce menstrual bleeding and provide birth control. An IUD works
by thinning the lining of the uterus so there is less to
shed during a period. The first couple of periods after
insertion may be heavy, but then they tend to lighten
or even go away completely. Be aware that the synthetic hormone can have adverse side effects such as

mood changes, weight gain, or skin changes for some women. Hormone-secreting IUDs have been associated with a small increase in breast cancer risk if used for longer than a year.

Surgical options for heavy bleeding or prolonged periods

Surgical alternatives such as hysterectomy or endometrial ablation are options for women who have tried other approaches without success. An endometrial ablation is the surgical destruction of the lining tissues of the uterus. This treatment is not a first-line therapy for heavy bleeding and should be considered only when medical and hormonal therapies have failed to control the bleeding.

A hysterectomy is the surgical removal of the uterus (with or without removal of the ovaries). It solves all the problems of bleeding but can create its own new set of issues to manage, especially if the ovaries are removed. Removal of the uterus can be life-changing, and often women are not warned about the consequences. For this reason, hysterectomy gets its own chapter later in this book.

Can I Still Get Pregnant?

Many women wonder about their fertility when they begin to experience irregular periods. It is important to remember that pregnancy can occur any time before menopause, even if a woman's periods are irregular. It is not uncommon during perimenopause to go months without a period, only to have it return. Eventually, levels are low enough to not stimulate the growth of the uterine lining; when this happens, periods stop.

Until this time, however, it is still possible to become pregnant. Current birth control recommendations in perimenopause suggest that if you reach menopause at 50 or before, you should continue with birth control for two years. If you reach menopause at 50–55, continue for one year. Of course, everyone is different, and you must make your own decision regarding method and timing in consultation with your doctor.

How to Live with Irregular Periods

Irregular periods are more of a nuisance than something that needs to be managed. They are a natural part of the perimenopause process. However, there are things you can do to support your body during this time.

Lifestyle changes

Lifestyle changes can help with irregular periods. Leading a sedentary lifestyle or consuming too much caffeine or alcohol can exacerbate symptoms. Increased stress can also increase the severity of irregular periods. Stress-relief techniques such as yoga or meditation can be helpful for this, as can simple die-

tary changes. Increasing the intake of complex carbohydrates, fruits, vegetables, fiber, and water can
help balance the hormones. Avoid foods and products that contain xenoestrogens such as soy, plastics,
pesticides, and cosmetics because they can alter estrogen levels.

Supplements

Supplements that target improvement of the proges-
terone/estrogen ratio can be helpful for normalizing
cycles. Chasteberry (also known as vitex agnus-
castus) is one supplement that is helpful, but it becomes less effective the closer a woman is to menopause. DIM (diindolylmethane) or IC3 (indole-3-
carbinol) both help lower estrogen levels and improve the balance of estrogen/progesterone. Bioidentical progesterone supplementation can also be
very effective if used in a cyclical manner. The goal
is not necessarily to completely normalize cycles, but
to control any symptoms that affect quality of life.

When to See a Doctor

It is perfectly normal during perimenopause to have
irregular periods. However, there are other conditions that can affect bleeding and warrant getting
checked out. If you've tried some of the tips above
with no success, it's time to see your doctor. Blood
clotting issues, fibroids, pregnancy, and occasionally
cancer are some of the reasons that might cause ab-

normal bleeding. Any bleeding after menopause should also be evaluated by your doctor.

Chapter 5:
Am I Going Crazy?

I sat down one morning recently, coffee in hand and opened my email. Like so many other days, I had a heartbreaking message in my inbox. It happens all the time. This is what Amy wrote to me:

"I'm embarrassed, I lost my job last month. I wasn't putting up my sales numbers. Truth is, I didn't have it in me. I lost my drive; that stubborn, energy-loving adrenaline rush that drove me for years to be a top performer and earn six figures. I feel like a failure. I understand that failing is OK, but the anxiety and emotions involved in all of this make no sense. I find myself waking up in the middle of the night with my heart racing, worrying about the most minor things. It's paralyzing and I wonder if it's all hormone related. It's like I'm the opposite person I was just 10 years ago. I decided to get my yoga 200-hour certification. I did it and I should be ecstatic, right? Nope, just glad I finished. I feel purposeless. To add to this, I was diagnosed at 41 with adult ADD. I think the mix of hormones, ADD, and anxiety is just too much. Will I ever feel like myself again?"

Perimenopause and Mental Health

The physical changes of perimenopause are challenging enough without throwing in a short but impactful list of mental health issues that can also arise. But it's important for all of us to bring this issue out of the shadows. We need to have open conversations about this transition and the link to mental illness rather than suffering in silence. Perimenopause affects not only our bodies, but our emotions and brain functionality. These symptoms can often be the most distressing changes in a woman's life because they can affect relationships, work life, the way a woman feels about herself, and her ability to handle the day-to-day stressors of life.

Depression, anxiety, mood swings, and panic attacks are very common in perimenopause and menopause, and they are most often related to—you guessed it—an imbalance between progesterone and estrogen. Hormones impact endorphin levels and neurotransmitters such as serotonin, dopamine, and GABA. So when estrogen and progesterone—the brain's neuromodulators—are up and down, so is your sense of well-being. Add to that life changes such as divorce, caring for aging parents, changing feelings about body image and your role in life, and/or substance abuse, and you have a recipe for a mental health disaster.

Perimenopausal Rage and Mood Swings

Angry outbursts may be the earliest sign of perimenopause and they can begin even before your cycle shortens. Nearly 40 percent of women have mood swings associated with hormonal changes that range from feelings of rage to intense PMS moodiness, anxiety, or despair. Women usually say this is different than what they have experienced before. It's totally new for them and pops up without warning. These are very obvious outbursts that involve over-reacting out of proportion to the situation at hand. It is extreme, emotional, hurts others, and often comes with feelings of regret.

These situations are very real for the thousands of "supermoms" and other modern women who have a thousand plates in the air all the time at work and at home. The rage I am talking about is one extreme example of an exaggerated PMS experience that many perimenopausal women have never experienced, and it surfaces for the first time ever in them. These types of outbursts are usually more common in the two weeks before a period.

Warning signs for perimenopausal rage

Mood swings within minutes

If you're fine one minute, and sad, overwhelmed, or crying the next, you may have a hormone imbalance. Moods that change like the flip of a light switch are a good clue.

Out-of-proportion anger

Totally overreacting to little things is part of this picture of rage. Agitation and irritability appear in response to minor events.

A long history of PMS

If you already have had a tendency toward PMS, the extreme hormone fluctuations of perimenopause can make this ten times worse. This is a situation where paying extra attention to good nutrition and stress management is critical.

Previous postpartum depression

Women who experience postpartum depression have brains that are wired to be very sensitive to hormone changes. Thus, they are more likely to be sensitive to the changes that come with perimenopause. This puts them at greater risk for developing more difficult perimenopausal and menopausal symptoms, including the above-mentioned perimenopausal rage.

What you can do to manage perimenopausal mental health concerns

Progesterone cream

Supplementing progesterone can be life-changing for some women who are struggling with the emotional aspects of perimenopause. It is not a one-size-fits-all option, but it is a low-risk option and works for many women. It is available over-the-counter. Progesterone is not the same as wild yam cream, so make sure to look for USP progesterone on the label. Progesterone usually works very quickly (within days), if it's going to be helpful, but I recommend giving it at least two cycles to assess response. If you suspect you have low cortisol (fatigue, salt cravings, depression, irritability), use with caution because it may increase feelings of anxiety and worsen insomnia.

Eliminate or reduce caffeine, alcohol and sugar

This nutritional approach is foundational for hormone balance. I have worked with many clients and have seen the positive changes that occur when sugar, caffeine, and alcohol are eliminated, and stress is well managed. All of these substances will exaggerate any hormonal symptoms that are occurring. Unstable blood sugar and an elevated stress response create a perfect storm for emotional outbursts and perimenopausal rage for women who are also experiencing hormone fluctuations.

Supplements

I prefer that my clients get most of their nutrients from food, but there are situations where medications (birth control pills, proton pump inhibitors) and/or stress can deplete vitamins and other nutrients. Some of my favorite all-purpose supplements are B-complex vitamins, magnesium, Vitamin D, and fish oil. I'll talk more in depth about these in my Foundational Five in Chapter 9.

Birth control pills

In general, I am not a fan of using birth control pills to manage perimenopause, but if you've tried other solutions and gotten no relief, then this is an option. The pill suppresses your normal hormone production, which in turn keeps your brain from being affected by the ups and downs of estrogen and progesterone. All birth control pills contain synthetic progestin and are associated with a slightly increased risk of breast cancer. They may also have other side effects such as weight gain.

Antidepressants

Antidepressants support the brain chemistry and help stabilize mood despite the hormone changes that are happening. With this support, your brain might better handle any wild hormone fluctuations that are wreaking havoc on your emotions during perimenopause, helping determine how you react to the triggers that result in rage. Antidepressants will not, however, solve any underlying hormone imbalances. My personal opinion is that they are overprescribed because it's easier to write a prescription than to get to the root cause of perimenopausal rage, but they certainly can play a role in a crisis situation while further exploration is going on relative to hormone imbalance.

There are various types and doses of antidepressants available by prescription from medical healthcare providers and psychiatrists. These will be discussed in detail in the depression section.

Addressing Anxiety in Perimenopause

You might be surprised at the number of women who mention anxiety as their most challenging symptom in perimenopause. And interestingly, this is completely new for many of them. Perimenopausal women suddenly feel unable to cope with situations that were never a problem before. Unrelenting anxiety can be frightening, and it can undermine confidence in a woman's ability to handle the day-to-day stressors of life. Many women assume they are slowly going crazy. The feeling of constant worry, tension, irritability, or loss of focus can be debilitating, especially if it results in scary things such as panic attacks or heart palpitations. Note: frequent episodes of heart rhythm irregularities should be checked out to make sure there's nothing more serious going on.

The good news about anxiety is that there is often a hormonal imbalance that can be corrected. Low estrogen or progesterone levels may be the culprit because both of these hormones have significant effects on the brain. The bad news is that you or your doctor may not recognize what's going on, and you may be dismissed with an "it's all in your head" diagnosis or come away with unnecessary prescriptions for antidepressants or anti-anxiety meds that do nothing to solve the underlying problem.

Fortunately, there are non-pharmaceutical approaches that can be helpful for anxiety. Because we are all different, responses may vary. Here are options to consider.

Supplements for anxiety

Ashwagandha

Ashwagandha is an adaptogenic herb that is often used as a natural remedy for anxiety because it helps to stabilize the body's response to stress. In addition to stabilizing cortisol, it protects the brain from degeneration and improves anxiety symptoms by destroying free radicals that cause damage to the brain and body. Ashwagandha helps to improve focus, reduce fatigue and fight anxiety without the side effects of most anti-anxiety medications.

Kava Root

Kava is used to improve mood, ease anxiety, and boost sociability. It works by stimulating the dopamine receptors. A randomized controlled trial conducted in Australia found that kava can be considered a first-line therapy for generalized anxiety disorder. Take kava under the guidance of your health care provider, as it can interact with certain medications such as benzodiazepines (Xanax, Ativan) or prescription sleeping pills (Ambien, Lunesta, etc.). Also, do not consume alcohol if you are using kava and be aware of the most common side effects, including headache, drowsiness, and diarrhea. There are reports of liver damage with kava, so it's wise to get baseline and periodic liver functions tests while taking it.

5-HTP (5-hydroxytryptophan)

Supplementing with 5-HTP, which is synthesized from tryptophan (an essential amino acid that acts as a mood regulator), can help to treat a number of issues that are associated with anxiety, including insomnia, moodiness, and headaches. 5-HTP increases serotonin, a calming neurotransmitter that transmits signals between the nerve cells and alters brain functions that regulate your mood and sleep patterns. The most common side effects with 5-HTP are nausea, vomiting, and diarrhea. Do not take it with any pre-scription anti-anxiety or antidepressant medications.

GABA (Gamma aminobutyric acid)

GABA is an inhibitory neurotransmitter that can cause a sedative effect, help regulate nerve cells, and calm anxiety. Anti-anxiety drugs such as Xanax and Valium work to increase the sensitivity of GABA receptors in the brain. GABA supplements are available in your local health food or vitamin store; another option is to use valerian root, which naturally increases your brain's GABA level and helps to calm anxiety.

Magnesium

Magnesium plays many important roles in the body, and magnesium deficiency is one of the leading deficiencies in adults. It is relaxing and helps GABA function, so if you're struggling with anxiety, you may want to try taking a magnesium supplement. Look for magnesium glycinate, taurate or threonate, which are forms that the body absorbs better. However, be aware that too much magnesium can cause diarrhea, so be careful with the dose.

B vitamins

B vitamins help to combat stress and stabilize your mood. Vitamin B6, in particular, serves as a natural remedy for anxiety because it works to boost mood, balance blood sugar levels, and maintain a healthy nervous system. Vitamin B12 is also important for fighting chronic stress, mood disorders, and depression. It helps to improve your concentration, improve energy levels and allow your nervous system to function properly. B vitamins can be depleted by medications such as birth control pills, estrogen, and proton pump inhibitors such as Nexium and Protonix.

Essential oils for anxiety

In addition to supplements, some essential oils can be very useful for managing anxiety. Lavender oil is relaxing and has been shown to reduce anxiety as effectively as benzodiazepines when used in an oral capsule (Lavela WS-1265).

Using lavender oil topically or inhaling lavender can help to induce calmness and relieve symptoms of anxiety such as nervousness, headaches, and muscle pain. Put three drops of lavender oil in your palm and rub it onto your neck, wrists, and temples. Dilute it in a carrier oil if you have sensitive skin. You can also diffuse lavender oil at home or at work, inhale it directly from the bottle for immediate relief, and add five to ten drops to warm bath water to fight anxiety naturally.

Roman chamomile essential oil is used to calm nerves and reduce anxiety because of its mild sedative and relaxation-promoting properties. Inhaling roman chamomile works as an emotional trigger because the fragrance travels directly to the brain to help fight anxiety symptoms. Diffuse five drops of Roman chamomile oil at home or at work, inhale it directly from the bottle, or apply it topically to the neck, chest, and wrists. Roman chamomile is also gentle enough for children to use as a natural remedy for anxiety.

Medications for anxiety

Pharmaceutical options for anxiety include benzodiazepines such as Xanax (alprazolam), Ativan (lorazepam), Klonopin (clonazepam), and Buspar (buspirone), a non-benzodiazepine alternative. The pharmacology of buspirone is not related to that of benzodiazepines, so it does not carry the risk of physical dependence and withdrawal symptoms for which those drug classes are known. Benzodiazepines have a high potential for dependence and can be difficult to stop if used long-term. In extreme cases, these may be helpful, but they don't solve the underlying problem. Having said that, short-term use can improve your ability to function while you're getting hormone imbalances sorted out.

Panic Disorder and Panic Attacks

A panic attack is the sudden onset of intense fear or discomfort that reaches a peak within minutes and includes at least four of the following symptoms:

- Palpitations, pounding heart, or accelerated heart rate
- Sweating
- Trembling or shaking
- Sensations of shortness of breath or smothering
- Feelings of choking
- Chest pain or discomfort
- Nausea or abdominal distress
- Feeling dizzy, unsteady, lightheaded, or faint

- Chills or heat sensations
- Paresthesia (numbness or tingling sensations)
- Feelings of unreality or being detached from your body
- Fear of losing control or "going crazy"
- Fear of dying

Some people experience what is referred to as "limited-symptom panic attacks," which are similar to full-blown panic attacks but consist of fewer than four symptoms.

Although anxiety is often accompanied by physical symptoms, such as a racing heart or knots in your stomach, the difference between anxiety and a panic attack is the intensity and duration of the symptoms. Panic attacks usually reach their peak level of intensity in 10 minutes or less and then begin to subside. But that 10 minutes can feel like an eternity. Because the symptoms tend to mimic those of heart disease, thyroid problems, breathing disorders, and other serious illnesses, people with panic disorder often make many visits to emergency rooms or doctors' offices, convinced they have a life-threatening issue.

Panic attacks can occur unexpectedly, regardless of whether you're in a calm or anxious state, and this is what really alarms women. It is not uncommon for individuals to experience a panic attack along with another psychological disorder. For example, someone with social anxiety disorder might have a panic attack before giving a talk at a conference.

Panic attacks are extremely unpleasant and can be frightening. As a result, people who experience repeated episodes often become worried about having another attack and may make changes to their lifestyle to avoid possible triggers.

Managing panic attacks

Cognitive behavioral therapy (CBT)

Cognitive behavioral therapy is considered to be the gold standard of treatment for panic attacks. CBT focuses on educating clients about their disorders; identifying and changing disordered thoughts and fears; teaching relaxation and other coping strategies; and helping clients face their fears. Research has shown that CBT for panic disorder is also effective when there are other emotional disorders present. The key component that makes CBT effective is the aspect of facing and accepting fears. This may sound counter-intuitive, but developing strategies to accept your emotional experience can be helpful during panic attacks because fighting against the experience engages the "fear of fear" cycle that can make things worse.

Breath work

Breath work is very helpful for panic attacks and anxiety. Effective breathing relaxes your autonomic nervous system and reduces episodes. Benefits of breathing exercises include:

- Their effect is nearly instant, and they work for almost everyone.
- They're not complicated
- They work to automatically slow your heart rate.

- They get you out of fight, flight, or freeze mode.
- You can do them anywhere.
- They're free.

Here are two breathing exercises you can try.

Abdominal breathing

Of all the breathing techniques for panic attacks and anxiety, this one is the best for self-calming. Here's how you do it:

1. Find a comfortable seated position.
2. Place one hand on your chest and one hand on your stomach.
3. Inhale deeply through your nose and use your lower hand to feel your diaphragm (not your chest) expand, drawing in air and inflating your lungs.
4. Take six to ten deep, slow breaths per minute for ten minutes each day.

Alternate nostril breathing

Alternate nostril breathing creates calm and balance and unites the brain's right and left sides.

1. Find a comfortable, seated position.
2. Hold your right thumb over your right nostril and inhale deeply through your left nostril.
3. At the peak of inhalation, hold your right ring finger over your left nostril and release and exhale through your right nostril.
4. Repeat the breaths three to five times.

Supplements and medications for panic attacks

The supplements and medications that are used to help with panic attacks are the same as those described previously for anxiety.

Other helpful approaches for panic disorder

In addition to other treatments, you may also find that the following can help with panic disorder:

- Yoga to relax your body and lower stress.
- Exercise to help calm your mind and offset potential side effects of medication such as weight gain.
- Avoiding alcoholic drinks, caffeine, smoking, and recreational drugs, which can trigger attacks.
- Getting enough sleep, so you don't feel draggy during the day.
- Acupuncture.

Depression

Signs of depression can include one or more of the following:

- Sadness
- Loss of energy
- Feelings of hopelessness or worthlessness
- Loss of enjoyment
- Difficulty concentrating
- Uncontrollable crying
- Difficulty making decisions
- Irritability

- Increased need for sleep, excessive sleep, or insomnia
- A change in appetite causing weight loss or gain
- Thoughts of death or suicide, or attempting suicide

Dr. Christiane Northrup, a well-known women's health expert, suggests in her book *The Wisdom of Menopause* that perimenopause is designed by nature to bring up the unfinished business of the first half of your life, so you can heal it and move on. Failure to do this increases the likelihood of full-blown depression, which is a well-known risk factor for heart disease, cancer, and osteoporosis. The women who are most likely to suffer the effects of hormonal swings and to have the most difficulty getting relief with hormone replacement are the same ones who have had mood problems during their earlier reproductive years and around childbirth.

As with many other symptoms of perimenopause, tackling depression requires a multi-faceted approach. Nutritionally, depression is often associated with low levels of vitamin D, so get your level checked. It should be between 50–80 ng/ml. Then, get out in the sunlight for at least 15 minutes a day without sunscreen, or start taking high dose vitamin D if it's low. You also need enough omega-3 fats (1–2 grams/day), because cell membranes are made up of omega-3 fats. These healthy fats are found in fish oil, salmon, olive oil, and ground flax seeds. Magnesium (400–800 mg day) is also very soothing for nerves.

Depression is associated with low levels of neurotransmitters such as serotonin and dopamine. The quickest way to raise those levels is to do things that are pleasurable. When you have fun, it raises nitric oxide levels in your blood, instantly raising your feel-good hormones. Exercise also lifts mild to moderate depression more than 50 percent of the time, so find forms of movement you enjoy and enlist your friends to join in. This will help keep you accountable and just makes the experience more fun.

You may also want to keep a journal. Pay attention to your dreams and record them along with your thoughts. Thought work can be especially helpful if you find yourself stuck in frequent spirals of negative thinking. One of my favorite ways to tackle negative thinking is to use a process called "The Work" by Byron Katie, which is a simple yet powerful process of inquiry that teaches you to identify and question the thoughts that cause your suffering. The process can be found online and is free; (www.thework.com/en).

Supplements for depression

B vitamins

B vitamins, especially folic acid and vitamin B6, can be helpful in mild depression. They can also increase the efficacy of prescription antidepressants. Be aware that folic acid can build up and cause an increase in anxiety, agitation and depression in individuals who carry the MTHFR genetic variant. If you have this (or aren't sure and want to be safe) use L-methylfolate instead of folic acid.

St. John's wort

St. John's wort is an herb that has long been used in Europe for mood disorders. Standardized extracts have shown an effectiveness equaling Prozac in the treatment of mild to moderate forms of the disease. It should not be taken with antiretroviral medications, birth control pills, or antidepressant medications (especially SSRIs such as Prozac or Celexa). Try 300 mg of an extract standardized to 0.3 percent hypericin three times a day. It takes about eight weeks to have a full effect.

SAMe (S-adenosyl-methionine)

SAMe has the advantage of working more quickly than St. John's wort. Use only the butanedisulfonate form in enteric-coated tablets, or in capsules. Try 400–1,600 mg a day on an empty stomach.

Saffron

This spice has been shown to be effective for depression, painful periods, and PMS. Two randomized trials have suggested that it is as effective as Prozac for depression at a dose of 15 mg twice a day.

Medications for depression

Medication can be an effective intervention for treating the symptoms of depression. The antidepressant you and your doctor choose often depends on your particular symptoms of depression, potential side effects, and other factors. As with medications for anxiety, antidepressants do nothing to solve an underlying hormone imbalance that may be causing depression.

Most antidepressants work by affecting chemicals in the brain known as neurotransmitters. The neurotransmitters serotonin, norepinephrine, and dopamine are associated with depression. How medications affect these neurotransmitters determines the class of antidepressants to which they belong.

Types of antidepressants

Selective serotonin reuptake inhibitors (SSRIs)

SSRIs are the most commonly prescribed type of antidepressant. They affect serotonin in the brain, and they're likely to have fewer side effects for most people. SSRIs can include citalopram (Celexa), escitalopram (Lexapro), fluoxetine (Prozac), paroxetine (Paxil), and sertraline (Zoloft).

Serotonin and norepinephrine reuptake inhibitors (SNRIs)

SNRIs are the second most commonly prescribed type of antidepressants. SNRIs can include duloxetine (Cymbalta), desvenlafaxine (Pristiq), levomilnacipran (Fetzima), and venlafaxine (Effexor).

Norepinephrine-dopamine reuptake inhibitors (NDRIs)

Bupropion (Wellbutrin) is the most commonly prescribed form of NDRI. It has fewer side effects than other antidepressants and is sometimes used to treat anxiety.

Tricyclic antidepressants

Tricyclics are known for causing more side effects (dry mouth, drowsiness) than other types of antidepressants, so they are unlikely to be prescribed unless there's a specific indication or other medications are ineffective. Examples include amitriptyline (Elavil), desipramine (Norpramin), doxepin (Sinequan), imipramine (Tofranil), nortriptyline (Pamelor), and protriptyline (Vivactil).

Monoamine oxidase inhibitors (MAOIs)

MAOIs have more serious side effects, so they are rarely prescribed unless other medications do not work. MAOIs have many interaction effects with foods and other medications, so people who take them may have to change their diet and other medications. MAOIs should not be combined with SSRIs or many other medications taken for mental illness.

A note on antidepressants

It's important to give your doctor regular feedback when you are taking an antidepressant, especially if you are prescribed any other medications. Keep track of your symptoms and any side effects that you experience. If you're having trouble finding a medication that works, genetic testing can help your doctor determine appropriate options.

Some antidepressants carry warnings that they may increase suicidal thoughts, particularly among young people. Be sure to let your doctor know if you experience any suicidal thoughts while on the medication. Above all, it's important to not get discouraged if an antidepressant isn't the right fit for you. Many women require a trial of more than one medication to get it right.

Never stop an antidepressant suddenly, otherwise adverse effects can occur. Antidepressant withdrawal is possible if you've been taking the medication longer than six weeks. Symptoms of this are sometimes called "antidepressant discontinuation syndrome" and typically last for a few weeks. Certain antidepressants (Paxil, Effexor) are more likely to cause withdrawal symptoms than others.

Stopping an antidepressant suddenly is likely to cause symptoms within a day or two. These include:

- Anxiety
- Insomnia or vivid dreams
- Headaches
- Dizziness
- Tiredness
- Irritability
- Flu-like symptoms, including achy muscles and chills
- Nausea
- Electric shock sensations
- Return of depression symptoms

To minimize the risk of antidepressant withdrawal, talk with your doctor before you stop taking an antidepressant. You will likely need to reduce the dose gradually over several weeks to allow your body to adapt.

The Darkest Side of Perimenopause

Janet was in her late 40s when we first began working together. She had just split up with her husband of one year and was a financially strapped single mom to two teenage boys. Janet had a long history of issues with depression, which culminated at age 42 with two hospitalizations for suicide attempts. While hospitalized, she was started on a number of mood-altering drugs. These stabilized her, but she knew deep down that something other than a chemical imbalance of neurotransmitters in her brain was to blame for her severe depression.

Janet decided to keep looking for answers on her own (while still taking her meds). She ultimately found a hormone clinic in a city about an hour from her home. Testing showed that she was severely depleted in estrogen, progesterone, and testosterone. Once she began therapy with hormone-impregnated pellets, the veil of her depression lifted, and she was eventually able to stop all of her medications.

Suicide risk in midlife is not something that is frequently talked about, but studies have shown that suicide rates are increasing. Middle-aged women between 45 and 64 had the highest suicide rate among women in both 1999 and 2014. This age group also had the largest increase in suicide rate between those years: a 63 percent increase from 6.0 to 9.8 per 100,000. It's probably no coincidence that those high numbers reflect the transition from vibrant baby boomers into middle and older age.

Suicide danger signs

The best way to minimize the risk of suicide is to know the risk factors and to recognize the warning signs of suicide. Take these signs seriously. Know how to respond to them. It could save someone's life. Warning signs that someone is considering suicide include a person who:

- says they want to die or kill themselves
- has a plan for killing themselves
- describes feelings of hopelessness and having no reason to live
- talks about feeling trapped or having unbearable pain
- talks about being a burden to others
- increases their use of alcohol or drugs
- exhibits reckless behavior or acts anxious or agitated
- sleeps too much or too little
- isolates themselves
- displays extreme mood swings

A suicidal person may not ask for help because they are not in an emotional position to reach out, but that doesn't mean that help isn't wanted. People who take their lives don't want to die, they just want to stop hurting. Suicide prevention starts with recognizing the warning signs and taking them seriously. If you think a friend or family member is considering suicide, you might be afraid to bring up the subject, but talking openly about suicidal thoughts and feelings can save a life.

Janet's case highlights the importance of making sure hormones are at least considered as a contributor to emotional problems in midlife. Seventy percent of women have no one to talk to about menopause. If your quality of life is significantly affected, don't suffer needlessly. Seek out the services of a licensed mental health professional to help you, and be sure it is someone with whom you can have an open line of communication and trust.

In our culture, mental health issues are often swept under the rug, making the path of least resistance (for women and their doctors) anything that will soothe us and make us feel better. This could be medication, or it could be any one of a number of numbing behaviors such as alcohol use, emotional eating, shopping, etc. Perhaps the question we should be asking ourselves in midlife is, "What is out of balance in my life that needs to be changed?" All the supplements or hormones in the world won't fix a life that needs a careful, honest look at what's going on. Emotional turmoil affects all aspects of brain function, and staying in situations that are distressing increases the likelihood of continued hormone imbalance and mental health issues.

Chapter 6:
Managing Your
Perimenopause Mindset

*"The biggest problem I've had since menopause is
lack of passion/interest/direction in my life."*
" I hate what I see when I look in the mirror."
"I feel frozen somehow."
"I seem to have lost myself."
*"I don't know what's normal and what's not. I focus
on every little thing about my body."*

Shift Your Mindset

The comments above are what I commonly hear
from my clients and the ladies in the Hormone Harmony Club. It's almost as if their bodies are conspir-
ing against them, and they don't know where to turn
or what to do. It's very easy to get stuck in mental
quicksand in midlife. But here's the danger of staying in that place: you get more of what you focus on.

It's easy to get caught up in negative thoughts
about aging, beauty, life purpose, and health (among

others). If you find yourself stuck in the muck of perimenopause, read on.

The beginning of the end or the start of something wonderful?

Perimenopause can either feel like the beginning of the end and something to wallow in, or it can be a time of creativity. It can also be an opportunity for reinvention when approached with a sense of curiosity about possibilities. It is vitally important to understand the power of the mind-body connection during this time. Many women leap from "solution" to "solution" looking for a magic bullet to cure the physical experiences they are having, when the true solution lies largely in managing their emotions and thoughts.

Carol Dweck, author of *Mindset*, describes two kinds of mindset: fixed and growth. The fixed mindset is focused on whether you will succeed or fail and is concerned about how you look to others. If you're stuck in the fixed mindset, you believe things will always be the way they are right now. A fixed mindset in perimenopause might include thoughts such as, "I could never give up sugar," and "I just have to suffer through." Women with a fixed mindset are much more likely to experience perimenopause as a negative time of their lives.

On the other hand, women with a growth mindset are eager for new challenges, knowing that their inner landscape, talents, and temperament can be cultivated. A growth mindset sets you up for lasting change. Adopting this way of thinking in perimenopause will lead you to being open to new possibilities and willing to make changes that will impact the way you feel physically and mentally.

If you're not familiar with mindset work, here's the bottom line: every belief we have about ourselves is a choice, and every thought we have is a choice. Changing thought patterns is hard work, but investing the time to practice cultivating a positive mindset will make a tremendous difference in your stress level and your experience of perimenopause. Let's start by looking at some of the common mindsets of perimenopausal women.

"I've been diagnosed with perimenopause."

It makes me crazy every time I hear a woman say she's been "diagnosed with perimenopause." Nothing about the menopause transition is an illness. It is a natural part of a woman's reproductive life. On one hand, having a diagnosis helps validate what you're experiencing and helps explain what's going on with your body; but on the other hand, attaching a diagnosis creates a certain level of powerlessness ("I can't help it, it's perimenopause") and increases the likelihood that you'll hyperfocus on every little twinge you feel in your body.

In today's world, the step that now comes after the doctor's "diagnosis" is a trip to the internet to Google perimenopause. And of course, this ramps up fear levels immediately when horror stories are at the top of the search page. It is one thing to educate yourself and quite another to further "diagnose" yourself with everything that can occur in perimenopause. Save your sanity. Find a few trusted resources to study and skip the deep dive that causes panic for many women.

Protect your DNA: "Who's that stranger in the mirror?"

In the Hormone Harmony Club, I regularly see comments such as this. *"I'm having mindset issues around the way my body is changing (thicker middle; loose, sheer skin on my face). I'm trying to stay positive and love my body—but there are days when I just feel ugly. I'm constantly comparing how I look to others in my age group. It makes me crazy."*

Nora Ephron was on to something when she wrote *I Feel Bad About My Neck*. This is a collection of short stories about midlife and the changes that happen. I have to be honest and tell you that the changes in my face are the hardest thing that I deal with physically. I have always looked younger than my age, but these days when I look in the mirror and see my neck, I feel old. All of the talk about wrinkles and lines equating to wisdom falls on deaf ears where I'm concerned.

Mindset challenges in perimenopause generally break down into thoughts we have about our physical body and emotional hurdles that we navigate. Let's take a look at each, along with the steps we can take to make the journey a positive experience.

Slowing the Aging Process

We can't stop the aging process. We can, however, manage the way we think about it and take steps to slow it down and keep our bodies as strong, healthy, and fit as long as possible. It's important to understand the process of aging and the things we do to ourselves that speed it up. One of the secrets of successful aging is keeping your telomeres long. What's a telomere, you ask? Telomeres are segments of DNA at the ends of our chromosomes. Think of them as the plastic tips of shoelaces that keep the ends of the laces together. Each time a cell divides, its telomeres become shorter. After years of splicing and dicing, telomeres become too short for more divisions. At this point, cells are unable to divide further, and they become inactive, die, or continue dividing anyway, an abnormal process that's potentially dangerous. Telomere length is the best marker of biological age, and the shorter your telomeres, the higher your risk of heart disease, obesity, cancer, stroke, dementia, and premature death.

Most of the forces that age us quickly and shorten our telomeres are well within our control: smoking, the sun, sugar, lack of sleep, stress, and sitting.

Smoking

Tobacco's effects on your overall life span are well-known. Smoking has been described by the World Health Organization as the single greatest preventable cause of disease, disability, and death globally. In fact, long-term smokers are robbed of as much as a decade of life, according to large-scale studies on both women and men. Tobacco smoke contains more than 3,800 different chemical components, many of which damage tissues directly or interfere with chemical processes necessary to keep those tissues healthy. The same chemicals can cause wrinkles and other premature aging of your skin.

Sun

"FRY NOW—PAY LATER!" These words of warning are from a skin cancer awareness advertising campaign by the American Academy of Dermatology, and they are the truth. I wish I'd known this back in the baby oil and iodine days when I was busy cooking myself despite not being blessed with any tanning genes. Your skin is like a scoreboard that starts keeping track the moment you are born. Every time we expose ourselves to the sun, changes to the skin occur. Over time, the look and feel of our skin changes.

Most people mistakenly think the changes in their skin are a normal part of aging. The fact is that the changes that we undergo (as a result of chronic UVA and UVB exposure) are preventable and are not part of the natural aging process. If your skin has not been exposed to UV radiation, it ages differently. Had too much sun in your lifetime? Here's what you might expect:

- A leathery skin texture
- Loose and wrinkled skin
- Dryness
- Freckles
- Sun spots (often seen on the backs of the hands, chest, shoulders, arms, and upper back, these are commonly referred to as liver spots, but they are strictly related to sun damage)
- Easy bruising
- Skin growths
- Rough/reddish skin patches (actinic keratoses)
- The appearance of red blood vessels
- Thinning and yellow discoloration of the skin

Cosmetic medical treatments can, to a certain extent, reverse the signs of skin aging, but understanding the harmful effects of the sun and modifying your habits are the keys to preventing further damage and should be the first steps towards rejuvenating your skin.

Sugar

Wrinkles, deep lines, and sagging skin are a partial byproduct of the process known as glycation, in which excess sugar molecules in the bloodstream attach themselves to collagen fibers in skin and ultimately cause them to lose their strength and flexibility. These bonds are called AGEs, or advanced glycosylation end products. High-glycemic index carbohydrates are rapidly converted to glucose in your bloodstream, which results in a loss of elasticity.

While wrinkled skin is one of the visible signs of AGEs, other degenerative diseases are also caused by glycation. These can be much more serious than wrinkles and include arterial stiffening, fatty deposits in blood vessels, cataracts, neurological impairment, diabetic complications...and the list goes on. AGEs lie at the very heart of the aging process.

Lack of sleep

Sleep-deprived women show signs of premature skin aging and a decrease in their skin's ability to recover after sun exposure. A study of 60 pre-menopausal women between the ages of 30 and 49 showed that the women who fell into the poor sleep category had more signs of skin aging, including fine lines, uneven pigmentation, and reduced skin elasticity. The researchers also found that those who enjoyed quality sleep were quicker to recover from stressors to the skin such as sun and environmental toxins. The classification of "poor sleep" was made on the basis of average duration of sleep and the Pittsburgh Sleep Quality Index, a standard questionnaire-based assessment of sleep quality.

Stress

Cultivating a less-stressful lifestyle promotes healthy aging in its own right, and it also sets the foundation for other habits that are important for successful aging. Stress management is so critical to managing perimenopause that it gets its own chapter later on in this book.

Sitting

Yes, sitting is the new smoking. Sitting is killing us. All the time we spend sitting in our cars or hunched over a keyboard is linked to increased risks of heart disease, diabetes, cancer, and even depression.

Here's what the research shows: sitting for more than three hours a day can cut two years off your life expectancy, even if you exercise regularly. And if you're vegging out in front of the TV for more than two hours a day, you lose another 1.4 years off your life. An Australian study showed that watching an hour of TV was about as lethal for anyone over 25 years of age as lighting up one cigarette.

Long periods of sitting cause changes in your body, which include:

Overproduction of insulin by your pancreas

Cells that aren't moving don't respond as well to the effects of insulin, so your body compensates by making *more* insulin, which can lead to diabetes over the long run. A study found that one extra hour of sedentary time a day was associated with a 22 percent increased risk for type 2 diabetes and a 39 percent increased risk for developing metabolic syndrome.

An increased risk for colon, breast, and endometrial cancers

The reason isn't clear, but one theory is that excess insulin encourages cell growth. Another theory is that regular movement boosts natural antioxidants that kill cell-damaging free radicals.

Poor circulation

Sitting decreases blood flow to your lower legs, putting you at risk for blood clots (DVT).

Mushy abs/glutes and tight hips

When you're standing, your abs hold you up, giving them a workout. If you're sitting, they don't have to do much. Same for your glutes. Hip flexors become tight if you're not upright, which can affect balance and increase your risk for falling.

Brain fog

Movement pumps blood to your brain, keeping you clear and energized. Perimenopausal women have enough issues with brain fog without adding to it.

Neck, back and shoulder strain

Craning your neck forward all day and slouching over a keyboard puts a lot of strain on your upper body. Wonder why you have those knots in your shoulder muscles? Look no further than the way you sit at a desk.

"I feel invisible"

Women often complain that they begin to feel invisible after a certain age. This doesn't mean men aren't interested, but by and large, society tends to ignore us. Unlike other cultures where the matriarch is revered and respected, ageism is alive and well in ours. As "women of a certain age," we need to call it out when we see it, but I believe feeling invisible is, to a certain extent, a choice.

If you feel invisible, this usually has more to do with your level of self-confidence than with age. I'm saying this from experience. When I was very young, I was painfully shy and did my best to keep from standing out in a crowd. I was not cute, athletic, or popular, so blending in was easy. It wasn't until I reached my 40s that I realized I wanted to step up my game. Working with a coach gave me the boost in self-confidence I needed and eventually I created my business at age 50. Now, as I approach 60, I feel better than ever both personally and professionally. If you feel as if you're melting into the woodwork, maybe it's time for a mindset reboot. Here's how you can achieve that:

Don't hide your age

Gone are our grandmothers' days when no self-respecting woman would dare share her real age. Twenty-nine and holding? No more. Own your age, openly, proudly, fearlessly.

Establish your personal style

Instead of following trends, now is the time to create your personal style. No matter how you dress, the important thing is that it is comfortable and reflects who you are today. If you feel like a queen in your clothes and accessories, you will always stand out.

Slay a goal

I did my first pull-up on April 16, 2014. I was 54 years old. That may not sound like a big deal, but most women can't do one at any age, much less at 54. I walked 60 miles in three days to raise money for breast cancer at age 51. I started my business when I was 50. We are capable of doing hard things. Doing something difficult when you're older really increases your self-esteem. So stretch yourself. Set a goal that feels out of reach, then slay it!

Surround yourself with likeminded people

My best friend is 74. She is a fiery redhead who does not look her age at all. I love her because she's fun, smart and caring and the only time I think about her age is on her birthday. When you make new friends, look beyond their age. Connect with people who share your same energy and joie de vivre. These like-minded ladies will always have eyes and ears for you.

"Who am I Now?"

"I believe that happiness is a choice no matter the trials and tribulations we are going through. I have chosen to embrace these changes and dive into finding things that bring me joy. For example, I had five

children and enjoyed raising them. Now they are all grown. So instead of focusing on the sadness of that, I decided that because I enjoyed my children so much, I would start watching a little one part-time to fill that void and give back to another child. Now I am venturing into my own interior design business, which gives me the ability to make my own hours and have flexibility and do something I have great passion for."

My client, Adrienne, who shared the story above, is making conscious choices to change how she approaches a possible loss of identity. Perimenopause can bring on the beginning of what feels like a "dark night of the soul." For women who don't take time to recognize what they do have choices about how to react when the going gets tough.

When I was 42, I struggled with almost every aspect of my life. I had a teenage daughter, a mother with cancer, a relatively new marriage, a good career (fortunately), a country club membership, and all the trappings of what looked to be the perfect life. But I was restless and bored, I had no idea where to turn next, and I made some really dumb decisions that cost me greatly. So I went to therapy and wandered through my "dark night." Then, at age 47, I found myself at a women's retreat, which began a period of deep self-exploration that continues even now. I hired a life coach, relocated despite my mother's illness, and began to put the pieces of my marriage back together. I survived and thrived and removed myself from the midlife quicksand that threatened to suck me under.

Stories like mine are all too common and I'm guessing many of my readers see bits of themselves in it. The struggle to "find" yourself in midlife is real. In the past, the major identity shift that women faced in midlife was the transition from motherhood to freedom. And while this is still part of the equation, we now have a generation of women who entered the workforce 40 years ago with more choices but few models for guidance.

Women today have high expectations of career advancement. Many in their 20s say, "I want to be CEO," then face the reality of having to live in the trenches for a while before they can even begin to rise up. As they enter their 30s and their career focus narrows, they seek meaningful, challenging work with opportunities to prove their value and make a significant contribution. This is where their experiences diverge from those of men. As women cope with the ongoing inequality in the workplace, #metoo issues, disappointments of dreams unmet, and continually feeling misunderstood and mismanaged, they begin to drop off the corporate ladder. Personal values and corporate values may clash, causing dis-ease and stress.

By the time they enter perimenopause and their 40s, many women have lost their taste for proving themselves. I know I did. When I first became a pharmacist, I said I wanted to be "semi-famous." I began collecting letters after my name, and I was on a mission to prove that I could do anything with a bachelor's degree in pharmacy. Telling me I couldn't do something was just the inspiration I needed to do "the thing." But by the time I was in my late 40s, I was D.O.N.E. I knew there had to be more.

Women aren't necessarily facing a midlife crisis. Instead, many are facing a midlife quest for identity.

Who are we if not mothers and career women (or whatever defined us in our earlier years)? If you are questioning what is next for your career and possibly your life, this is a great time to reach out to friends who might be going through a similar experience. One of the worst things busy women do is put their friendships on the back burner. There is no need to tough it out on your own. Find a friend who is also interested in personal development who won't judge the struggle you are experiencing. A good coach can help as well.

Here are some questions you might explore:

- What do I feel I should have done by this time in my life?
- Is there something more important and fulfilling that I can focus on now?
- What do I want more of in my life? What is asking to be set free?

Above all, don't let people tell you that you should be perfectly happy with your life. It is OK to lose your equilibrium when others think your life should be smooth sailing. It is OK to question your life's purpose. It is OK to say, "I don't know who I am." And it is better to ask the questions and seek the answers than to live a numb life that ends in regret.

And Now for the Bright Side

Perimenopause definitely brings challenges for creating and maintaining a healthy, positive mindset. But there are some gifts that come with it.

The "disease to please" is cured

Many of us were raised to always put others first and to be seen and not heard. *Don't make a scene, give adults your seat, play quietly in your room during the cocktail party, don't impose on others by asking for help, don't order the most expensive thing on the menu*...these are just a few of the early messages I got in my family. All of these discouraged me from ensuring my own needs were met and encouraged me to stay small and quiet, which I dutifully did. Then, when we marry and have children, we focus on the needs of the family while we remain at the bottom of the priority list. All this people-pleasing sets us up for overwhelm and generally feeling pissed off. When you spend all of your time going out of your way to please others, it's very difficult to get what you want from your own relationships, which leads to anger, frustration, and sadness that gets buried in your body. This creates a situation of chronic stress, and you can bet that it will show up as a physical manifestation such as weight gain, insomnia, or depression.

But here's the gift. As estrogen levels fall through perimenopause, so does the tolerance for people-pleasing and putting up with loads of B.S. I promise that by the time you hit menopause, you will no longer give a rat's ass about what anyone thinks of you.

Your prescription for the disease to please

The perimenopause years are an excellent time to begin to cure yourself of people- pleasing. The hormonal drops that help with this cure will take care of themselves, but the rest is up to you. And it takes practice.

Start by looking at your priorities. Ask yourself what you need most right now. It can be simple: maybe you need more sleep or to make better food choices. Maybe you need to say "no" more often, or you need more help around the house. Whatever it is, pick just one thing to work on.

Let's take getting some help around the house as an example. When my daughter was 10, I bought her an alarm clock, showed her how to work the washer and dryer and where she could find stuff to make lunch for school. It then became her job to get herself out of bed and ready for the school bus, lunch in hand. She assured me I was the meanest mother ever. But I had enough on my plate without having to be responsible for tasks she could easily do. I know that part of success here depends on the kind of kid you have, but if you set expectations (and let them fail a couple of times) they will usually step up to the plate.

My point is this. You don't get extra points for trying to do everything yourself. Ask for help. The able-bodied members of your household need to pitch in and do their share. Once you get the first changes down, move on. Ask for favors. Say no to one thing a week. And notice how you feel when you do these things. If you think people are thinking badly of you, here is the truth: they are not. Instead, they are moving on to the next person they know who is not a recovering people-pleaser.

A call to creativity

If you've been so focused on work and family that you haven't had a chance to tap into your creative side, midlife may be the time to do so. There's a myth that people are either born creative or not, and that creative people have something extra that the rest of us don't have. I've always said my sister was born with the creative genes. She was an excellent painter in her younger years, and I couldn't draw a stick figure. But the truth is that I had other creative abilities—such as writing a book. Creativity is nothing more than the ability to make new things or think of new ideas. We are all born creative, but by the time we reach adulthood, creativity has been "educated" out of many of us by schools, society, and business. Our job in midlife is to get it back.

Why does creativity come alive in midlife? Psychologist Kathleen Brehony says that two important things happen in midlife: first, we experience a heightened awareness of death; and second, we ultimately recognize that our own time is limited and that we'd better get on with it. As she says, "The deepest inner strivings of the soul press for expression," and so paradoxically, the fear of death and the urge to leave a legacy can bring us alive in creative new ways at midlife.

Creativity comes in many forms. Many of us may think of artists or writers when it comes to creative people. But how about inventors or entrepreneurs? That's creativity too. If you are feeling as if there is something that wants to come out of you, seize the moment and trust your instinct. Don't overthink it—try on your inspired ideas.

One way to cultivate creativity is to write out your ideas and tell them to friends. I keep a small journal in my purse so I can capture random thoughts as they come up. My tiny purple notebook goes everywhere with me. Julia Cameron, author of *It's Never Too Late to Begin Again* and *The Artist's Way*, has Morning Pages, a practice of writing three free-form pages, first thing, every morning. Using this practice can be really helpful in focusing diffuse creative thoughts.

Escaping the Midlife Mindset Muck

If you're swirling around in the muck of your mindset, there are ways to break free. Some are easy, and some take practice.

Let go of your previous expectations

Your married life may be changing (or gone completely), your job or business is not making you happy anymore, your kids are almost grown or have left home and aren't asking you where their socks are anymore, and it's time for you to let go. It may also be time to redefine what your job is giving you and ask for more. I'm not just talking money here (although there's nothing wrong with that). I'm talking fulfilment, enjoyment, camaraderie, and recognition. If this means having to find a better gig, so be it. Ask yourself just one question, "What do I want?"

Declutter (both people and stuff)

A few years after I'd gotten out of college, I got a call from my mom. She told me I had two weeks to come get what I wanted out of her attic or it was going to the curb. That attic had been the personal storage facility for my sister and me, but now the purge was on. I couldn't understand what was so urgent about this at the time, but now I get it. Completely. We keep all our kids' school stuff, our family photos, and other important things—but there comes a time when we need to give them to the people they belong to. I've done this with my daughter as well.

Decluttering is a powerful process. Clutter is the stuff that no longer serves us. It fills up our space (mentally and physically). One of the basic tenets of feng shui, which is the ancient art of creating a harmonious environment in your home, is that clutter represents stagnant energy. In order for energy to flow and create a space that feels like a peaceful sanctuary, the clutter must be cleared.

Just as clutter keeps energy stagnant, it can also keep other areas of your life stuck. Do you avoid having friends over because your home is not in order? Have you put off planning a vacation or starting a new project because your life feels too out of control? Does a lack of organization make daily tasks, such as paying bills or putting away groceries, difficult? If so, let the stuff go. It doesn't have to be overwhelming. Pick one area to start with, preferably one that doesn't contain a lot items that you're attached to, set a timer and work until the timer goes off. Thirty minutes is a really good place to start.

As you move through the space, ask yourself three questions about each item. Do I love it? Do I need it? Do I use it? If the answer is no to all three questions, out it goes. Sort your discard pile into broad categories (trash, recycle, or donate). Allow the feelings or emotions that are attached to an item to surface. Acknowledge them...and continue moving on. Take the things you want to get rid of out of the house ASAP. The longer things sit around, the more likely it is they'll find their way back into your home.

Give yourself permission to walk away when the time is up. Repeat these steps until your space feels open, peaceful, and beautiful. If you're having trouble tossing stuff, ask a friend to help. Having an impartial person around can help you be more objective.

As an aside, we sometimes need to declutter or detox the people in our lives as well. If you have relationships that are sapping your energy or that feel very one-way, it may be time to let them go, too.

Start a gratitude journal

We all have something to be grateful for every day. If you are spending your mental energy looking for those things on a daily basis, you have less time to focus on what's going wrong. Try writing down five things you're grateful for at the end of each day. This simple exercise can really shift your perspective.

Get outside

There are two great reasons to do this. First, sunlight greatly enhances your feeling of well-being (and gives your vitamin D levels a boost). Second, a number of studies have documented the positive effects that being in nature can have on mood. Spending as little as five minutes a day connecting with the outdoors helps.

Take the first step (not the first ten)

Want to lose 10 pounds? Start with the first pound. Exercise? Start with five minutes once a week. That may sound so small that you think, "Why bother?" But your goal is to create momentum, and small successes are the key to achieving that.

Relax

Set aside a few minutes every day for an intentional time out. Do some deep breathing, meditation, or yoga. Take a nap. Sometimes when we're stuck in our gunk, we're just plain tired. It's OK to wave the white flag and care for your body.

Put your worries in a box

If you're prone to anxiety and worrying about every ache or pain, give yourself a specific, limited time for this. Here's what I mean. Schedule your worry time daily. Say from 8–8:15 a.m. For that 15 minutes you get to worry about everything on your list. Go big!

Because at 8:15, you're done for the day. Another way to do this is to get a decorative box and make it your worry box. Write down what you're worried/anxious about, put it in the box, and turn it over to whatever higher power you believe in. Consider it handled.

Reach out

Surround yourself with friends who love and support you. Find a live or virtual community of women who are traveling this same road as you are, and become a part of that community. It's incredibly helpful when you discover that what you are experiencing is common and that you are not alone. That single realization can be a game-changer for many women. That's what my Hormone Harmony Club (www.drannagarrett.com/hhc) is all about.

Perimenopause can be a challenging time of life. But it can also be a time of great awakening if you allow it. If you're feeling stuck, give yourself grace, and know that this too will pass.

Chapter 7:
Navigating Relationships:
From the Boardroom to
the Bedroom

Katie found her Prince Charming later in life. They married when she was 39, and because they both had known fertility issues, they headed straight to a fertility clinic after saying "I do." The clock was ticking and they both desperately wanted children. Two cycles of IVF later, they were joyfully pregnant.

Katie gave birth to a beautiful daughter, but instead of settling into the joy of mommy-hood, she went straight into perimenopause, which for her manifested as panic attacks and anxiety in the second half of her cycle. When her maternity leave ended, she dragged herself back to a stressful job working for a hedge fund in New York City and began navigating the logistics of daycare and breastfeeding as a working mom. Unfortunately, her panic and anxiety finally won the battle, and she was forced to leave her job because she couldn't handle the day-to-day pressure.

Katie took some time to regroup and decided to give work life a try again on a part-time basis. One day, as she was driving to work, her heartbeat went crazy. She could feel the fear rising in her throat as she gripped the steering wheel. Could she make it to work? Should she pull over and call 911? Waves of panic swept over her, and she decided to try to make it to the office. Katie tried to rationalize it as just another panic attack, but something about it felt different. She made it to the bank and asked her colleagues to call 911. Because panic attacks and anxiety were her norm (and they all knew it), no one called. Finally, she drove herself to the hospital where she was found to be in atrial fibrillation, a kind of irregular heart rhythm. She stayed in this rhythm for seven hours, right up until the time she was scheduled to have it shocked back into a normal beat. Fortunately, the rhythm corrected itself right before the procedure.

As with previous episodes, she noticed that it was the end of her period and began to wonder whether this could be related to perimenopause and a hormone imbalance, but none of the medical professionals she saw during the entire ordeal were willing to test her hormones. Katie lasted a few more weeks at the bank before she was fired. Now she is on disability, and her family is in danger of losing their home and everything they've worked hard to build.

Perimenopause at Work

When I began to think about this chapter, I asked the ladies in the Hormone Harmony Club to share their experiences of how perimenopause has affected their work life. I couldn't believe the responses I got (including the story above) and how broad the range of experiences was. They covered it all: from snarky male bosses who made jokes at their female employee's expense, to job loss because of being unable to function, to soiled clothing due to flooding in meetings. None of this is what we want for our Savvy Sisters.

The topics of perimenopause and menopause are not common water cooler talk in most workplaces. We talk about pregnancy, breastfeeding, and cancer, but perimenopause is off the table. Women don't want anyone to know that they are affected by it, and men don't want to hear about it. But here's the thing: every woman goes through it in one way or another. That means 27 million people who are working in all kinds of jobs are dealing with it right now.

If you look at research regarding the effects of the menopause transition on work life, the UK is light years ahead of the US in research on this topic. A British survey found that 20 percent of women believe that menopause has had negative impacts on their managers' and colleagues' perceptions of their competence, and so most women remain silent about it.

In another study, researchers at the University of Nottingham in the UK found that many women were hesitant to disclose menopause-related problems to their manager, particularly if the manager was younger than them and/or male. Of the women who took time off from work due to perimenopausal or menopausal symptoms, only half of them disclosed the real reason they were absent. Some women in the study considered working part-time, but they were afraid this would have a negative impact on their career. More than half of the women in the study said they were unable to negotiate flexible work arrangements when dealing with symptoms.

As you might imagine, perimenopause is not on most employers' agendas. In fact, I know of no perimenopause or menopause-specific health and well-being policies that exist in the United States. In the UK, organizations are ahead of the curve, and some companies have instituted training programs for managers and employees. Creating policies around perimenopause and menopause is a double-edged sword. Women don't want to be singled out as not being able to perform their jobs with the same level of competence as younger women, but many could be helped if there was some flexibility with working arrangements. Finding the balance between harm and help is critical to keeping midlife women in the workplace.

In my mind, this issue is similar to pregnancy and maternity. Imagine a woman in her early 30s telling her manager she is pregnant. Celebration all around! Her job is protected for up to 12 weeks using the Family Medical Leave Act (FMLA) in the US. Now imagine the same woman, 20 years later, telling the same manager she is experiencing severe insomnia, hot flashes, and night sweats, and she wants to work from home when these symptoms are especially problematic. The evidence suggests that, even if this woman felt comfortable talking to her boss about this (and many, many midlife women workers do not), she is likely to be met with a shrug of the shoulders at best. Can't handle your responsibilities?

Sorry, guess you'll have to look elsewhere. There's no protection for this midlife woman.

Research has shown that the more frequently women reported experiencing perimenopause-related symptoms and the more bothersome the symptoms, the more likely they were to feel less engaged at work, less satisfied with their jobs, more inclined to quit their jobs, and less committed to their employment. Studies have shown that perimenopause symptoms can also have a significant impact on attendance and performance in the workplace, with some women being misdiagnosed as suffering from mental health or other conditions. This impact on a woman's work can be wrongly identified as a performance issue. In fact, I met a woman from the UK who had a high-level job in human resources who had such bad brain fog that she ended up quitting her job—and she had no clue what was going on. She is now an advocate for teaching line managers and employees about the menopause transition and its impact in the workplace through her company, Simply Hormones (www.simplyhormones.com).

How employers can support their staff

On the employer side, early recognition, education, and appropriate accommodations can help prevent perimenopause-related absenteeism. If perimenopause and menopause were brought out into the light instead of being whispered about, women would have a safe space to talk about their concerns with their work colleagues and managers. Part of my goal as a speaker and author is to help teach organizations how to create an empathetic and caring environment so women know what is going on with their bodies and feel comfortable talking about it. Here are some ways I believe employers can better serve the needs of women in midlife.

Be flexible

If your employee discusses her perimenopause symptoms with you and asks for accommodations, such as the ability to work from home some days, be as open as possible. Communicate understanding and make allowances as long as they don't interfere with the quality of your employee's work.

Educate management and employees

Employers can work to change the culture and stigma around a normal event that all women will experience. Some ways to educate employees may include holding awareness events or scheduling group wellness classes.

Be aware of legalities concerning symptoms of menopause

While there are no specific laws governing the treatment of perimenopausal or menopausal women, actions that arise as a result of symptoms could be classified as age or sex discrimination. It's important for an employer to be able to recognize what behaviors might be the result of hormonal changes, as opposed to poor performance. Simply being aware of the challenges associated with this transition can help an employer gauge what may or may not be the result of perimenopause.

When Perimenopause Meets Middle School

Lisa is in a tailspin. For the third morning in a row, her daughter, Meredith, is screaming at her at the breakfast table. As Meredith rages, Lisa wants nothing more than to lay her head on the table and cover her ears, but instead she allows herself to become an actor in the unfolding drama, and soon the two of them are having a world class battle.

Lisa is just entering the throes of perimenopause. Sleepless nights, hideous mood swings, crying jags at odd times, and crushing fatigue are making her life hell. And now this little cherry on top? She wonders where it all went wrong. Why her once-darling seventh-grade daughter is now a ticking time bomb most days. Meredith is prone to go off about anything and nothing on a moment's notice, and Lisa has no idea what to do.

Lisa and Meredith are at the hormonal intersection of perimenopause and middle school. As if the highs, lows, and hair-pulling frustrations of raising a hormonal teenage girl weren't enough, more and more mothers are wading through this turbulent time during their own hormonal journeys: perimenopause and menopause. And it's not pretty.

Many women of our generation postponed having children until relatively late in life, so they could build careers. In fact, according to the National Center for Health Statistics, the birth rate for women ages 35 through 39 rose steadily from 1979 to 2007 (though that number has slipped some since). Meanwhile, the birthrate in 2013 (the latest data available) for women ages 40 through 44 was 10.4 births per 1,000 women, the highest rate reported in more than three decades.

If you had a daughter in your 30s, there's a really good chance your hormonal chaos will collide with hers. Most children enter puberty between the ages of 11 and 15, with some making the big change between their eighth and ninth birthdays. Typically, girls enter puberty about 18 months earlier than their male counterparts. So if you had her when you were 30 and she entered puberty when she was 12, you would be 42. This math equation lands you smack in the average age of entering perimenopause.

Like Lisa, you may be at a loss for ways to deal with this. The first step is to do some research. As the parent, it's up to you to navigate this storm, even when you don't feel like it. Understanding that the two of you are going through many of the same emotional swings can be really helpful in bringing peace to your home. Both of you are having huge shifts in hormonal levels (in girls, estrogen levels increase eight-fold during puberty).

Want to dial down the drama? Here are some survival tips for days when it feels as if you and your little darling are turning the family upside down.

Keep the lines of communication open

Have an honest talk with your daughter about what's going on with you. Let her know you can relate to what she's experiencing. As a bonus, know that she will thank you later when she hits perimenopause.

Empathize

Recognize that even though you were a teenager once, chances are you didn't have to deal with the kinds of pressure today's kids experience. Yes, we dealt with mean girls and cliques. But no one could bash you on social media. Getting into college was not the anxiety-producing experience that it is now. We weren't overscheduled and under-rested. Today's teens report much higher levels of anxiety and stress than our generation did.

Be quick to call a time-out

When an argument starts to spiral out of control and you sense you may say things you'll regret, walk away and cool off. Revisit the issue later when everyone's had a chance to calm down.

Check your stress level

The physical symptoms you're experiencing combined with the day-to-day stress of work and home life can be recipe for a short fuse. Figure out what your top three priorities are and consider letting the rest go. Your sanity will thank you for this.

Remember, this is a season and it will pass

The hormonal chaos will eventually die down for both of you, and if you can keep a sense of humor, your relationship will survive and thrive.

Get support!

If your home has become too much of a battlefield to deal with effectively, it may be time to enlist professional help. It's possible that something bigger is going on with your child than hormone shifts, and family therapy may be the answer you're looking for. If finances are an issue, there are many community resources you may be able to access for help.

In Lisa's case, she decided her best approach was to start by controlling her symptoms, so she could be less reactive. We worked together to test her hormones and re-engineered her lifestyle to help bring her body into better balance. I also helped her create some strategies to manage stress and say yes less frequently so that she could focus on herself and her relationships.

Not everyone's symptoms or experiences are the same, and no magic solution exists. But as more women find themselves in hormone hell, it's good to know that there are options to avoid at least some of the fireworks—our own, anyway. Because as far as I know, teenage drama is here to stay!

Perimenopause in the Bedroom

Jennifer is doing a mental eye roll. Her husband, Adam, is once again trying to tell her how she should be managing her newly acquired brain fog and forgetfulness. Up until this point, Jennifer has been a world-class multi-tasker, but these days, it feels as if she forgets as much as she remembers. "Leave sticky notes for yourself and set an alarm on your phone to remember to get the kids," he suggests. "Maybe you should get checked for Alzheimer's. You know it runs in your family." Jennifer wants to smack him. She knows her brain fog is related to perimenopause and her out-of-balance hormones. She's tried to talk to Adam about it, but he has no time for her or interest in what she's saying. So the mansplaining continues.

"I don't need him to fix me!" she tells me. "I just want him to listen and try to understand that I'm doing the best I can."

This is a sentiment I hear a lot in my Hormone Harmony Club. I recently asked these ladies what their biggest challenges are when it comes to dealing with partners and perimenopause. As you might expect, the responses were plentiful and varied. What surprised me was the number of women who live with partners who had incredibly selfish reactions to the whole process...which manifested as "get over it," or "I'll leave if things don't change quickly." One woman posted that verbal abuse is much harder to deal with in perimenopause. As if anyone should put up with that at *any* point in their marriage.

It is no secret that navigating relationships in perimenopause and menopause can be tricky. Midlife is a time when women begin to reflect on what they want for themselves and worry less about what others think. Now is the time to take a good hard look in the darker corners of your relationship. Your emotional and physical health depend on it. Stresses and unresolved relationship issues that boil just below the surface will manifest somewhere, usually in the form of illness. We're not meant to have the same relationship with our partner that we did in our 20s or 30s, so it may be time renegotiate the sacred contracts we made long ago.

Men need to understand perimenopause too. If it's hard for you to understand the changes, imagine what it must be like for the partners who navigate this time with us. My experience has been that men (at least the man I'm married to) aren't excited about the idea of their relationship changing. Every time I've stepped up into something bigger in my life, I've gotten pushback. Is that because my husband doesn't want me to be successful and happy? No, it's because he's scared of what might change.

Perimenopause can be a lonely place. Your body is changing, your emotions are all over the map, and sometimes you just feel like curling into the fetal position for the next five years. And the loneliness only intensifies if you can't talk about what's going on with the people you love most. You may have tried to talk to your partner or husband about it, and while he or she is understanding (to a point), it's hard to get it when he or she is not walking in your shoes, especially if you are not 100 percent sure what's going on. And even though this is a "woman's issue," the impact it can have on a marriage can quickly turn it into a couple and/or family issue, too.

Divorce that is initiated by women is more common than ever before, and in many of those cases, the women filing are in their 40s, 50s, and 60s. According to Dr. Christiane Northrup, the hormonal changes that occur can result in women placing their marriages under a proverbial microscope, with the likelihood that instances of inequality, problems in the marriage, or ways their own needs aren't being met will be noticed like never before. And remember curing the "disease to please" that I talked about earlier? The family is the first place where the "cure" lands. Women go from putting others' needs first to becoming more aware of their own needs and wants. This alone is enough to change the status quo of many marriages.

So the question is this: how do you renegotiate this transition as partners rather than ending up as adversaries? First, you need to be clear on what you need and want. Many women never allow themselves the luxury of asking this question. But if you can't clearly state what you need, you can't expect your partner to understand. Mindreading is rarely anyone's forte.

Next, have an open, honest conversation. Assume your partner has no clue what perimenopause is all about, and be prepared to describe the process and all that goes with it. Use "I" vs. "you" statements (this is a good idea for all tough conversations). Here's an example: compare "You never say thank you for anything I do around the house!" with "I don't feel valued when I never get a thank you for what I do around here." See how different those two statements feel? Ask for what you need and acknowledge your role in any of the bumpiness the two of you may be experiencing. Let's face it, when riding the hormonal highs and lows of perimenopause, we can say and do some pretty hurtful things. Sometimes they shock even us. Let your partner know you're sorry and you're doing the best you can.

Then, give your partner time to process your conversation. I know in my own relationship, this is a crucial step. Be prepared to revisit your "asks" as needed.

And if your partner is a selfish ass hat?

Sometimes all the talking and negotiating in the world won't budge someone who truly doesn't care about your needs. While a thorough discussion of divorce is beyond the scope of this book, you may need to consider that option, especially if there is verbal or physical abuse involved. Leaving a long-term relationship can be scary in midlife, but in my personal opinion, it's not nearly as scary as spending the rest of your life with an uncaring, selfish person. You deserve better. Go get it.

Chapter 8:
Managing Stress:
The Key to the Kingdom
of Hormone Balance

I once coached a brilliant nurse named Jackie who had a potato chip problem. In every aspect of her food life, she made amazing, healthy, nourishing choices. Until she was on her drive home from work. It was as if her car had a mind of its own, and every day, she'd whip into the grocery store parking lot and run in to buy a bag of chips. Jackie was in graduate school, and when she finally sat down at night to study, out would come the bag of chips. She'd nibble on the first one as she started her work. Eventually, the scene would devolve into a mindless hand-to-mouth, salty, crunchy, chip fiesta. And she'd eat the whole bag.

Jackie couldn't understand what was wrong with her. Actually, nothing was "wrong." What we finally discovered in our work was that those potato chips were her crunchy stress-management strategy for a life that had basically been stripped of everything else she found pleasurable. Between work, school, and marriage, there wasn't a second left for enjoy-

ment of anything except those chips. My client was a very high achiever and was driven to get As on everything. Once she was able to see that there was really no need to get As in grad school (except to satisfy her inner perfectionist), she stopped grinding away and opened up some space for ballroom dancing, something that had previously brought her joy. And once she began dancing again, the need for the chips evaporated.

Stress is Killing Us

We've already established that some women experience particularly severe symptoms when they go through their perimenopausal years. But why is there so much variation from one woman to another? Lifestyle choices play a big role, but in my opinion, the biggest culprit is stress. Consider the following:

- Forty-three percent of all adults suffer adverse health effects from stress.
- Seventy-five to ninety percent of all doctor's office visits are for stress-related ailments and complaints.
- Stress can play a part in problems such as headaches, high blood pressure, heart problems, diabetes, skin conditions, asthma, arthritis, depression, and anxiety.
- The Occupational Safety and Health Administration (OSHA) declared stress a workplace hazard. Stress costs American industry more than $300 billion annually.

- The lifetime prevalence of an emotional disorder is more than fifty percent, often due to chronic, untreated stress reactions.

Stress hormones and sex hormones share a common thread: the raw materials that make your stress hormones happen to be the same chemicals that make your sex hormones. The body triages its needs, and its safety is the number one concern. Your body will always make stress hormones (cortisol, epinephrine and norepinephrine) first, at the expense of other hormones. This is exactly what is supposed to happen. When your body is under attack from a real or imagined threat, stress hormones will make your vision sharper, increase your mental acuity, and increase your blood sugar for energy so you can run from danger. When the system is operating correctly, your stress hormone levels fall once the immediate threat is gone.

Unfortunately, the price of all this stress is chronically high levels of cortisol, which results in decreased immune function, decreased liver function, hormone imbalance, decreased fertility, and slowed gastrointestinal function. Ultimately, cortisol causes breakdown all over the body and may result in chronic diseases such as diabetes, depression, digestive problems, and even cancer.

Stress affects everyone differently. It's mostly a matter of perception. Some people thrive on a fast-paced lifestyle and can effortlessly bounce from task to task. For others, that pace creates a constant state of overwhelm. The goal isn't to entirely rid ourselves of stress, however. First, because stress is unavoidable in our world today; and second, because without it, life would be pretty dull. Instead, the key is to channel the energy that stress creates into productive action in a way that feels balanced and good.

Many of us live in such a way that we no longer recognize when we are stressed. Our society has created the impression that living in hyperdrive is just what we're supposed to do. But our bodies think otherwise. You may say you're not stressed, but your body knows your truth. And the key to bringing everything back into balance is to convince the body and your nervous system that your world is safe.

Understanding your nervous system

Your autonomic nervous system (which works involuntarily) has two main components: the sympathetic and the parasympathetic systems. The sympathetic nervous system prepares the body to react to stresses such as threat or injury, causing your muscles to contract and your heart rate to increase. It is responsible for the "fight, flight or freeze" responses. The parasympathetic nervous system is the part of the autonomic nervous system that controls functions of the body at rest ("rest and digest"). It helps maintain balanced systems in the body, causing your muscles to relax and your heart rate to decrease. The two systems generally do not play well together. Knowing this, it's easy to see how balance in the body can get wildly off track when the sympathetic system is running the show. If you are faced with immediate danger, the body will divert blood flow from parasympathetic nerve functions (such as digestion) to sympathetic nerve functions (such as muscle contraction and heavy breathing to run away). And when your body thinks you're under constant attack, the parasympathetic system never has a chance to take over the reins.

The upside of stress

Too much stress is bad for us, but when the body is responding in a good way to acute stressful events, it can be a plus. We need those powerful fight-or-flight hormones our bodies produce when we're about to be run over by a bus or when confronted with an unexpected, needed-it-yesterday deadline at work. Short-term (lasting for less than 24 hours) stress also triggers the production of protective chemicals and increases the activity in immune cells that boost your body's defenses. Studies suggest that this surge makes vaccinations more effective and may even protect against certain types of cancer. Small amounts of stress hormones can also help make your memory sharper. In 2009, researchers from the State University of New York at Buffalo found that when rats were stressed by being forced to swim, they remembered their way through mazes far better than more relaxed rats did.

The key, of course, is balance. Too little stress makes you bored and unmotivated. Too much, and you become not just grouchy, but sick. It's important to pay attention to your body's stress meter to keep it from heading into the danger zone. Mental fogginess, frequent colds, and increased sensitivity to aches and pains are all signs of an overwhelmed immune system. Autoimmune diseases such as psoriasis, rheumatoid arthritis, and inflammatory bowel disease may flare up. If you find yourself crossing the line into negative stress, there are strategies you can use to manage it. We'll get into more about this later.

The cortisol connection to sex hormones

We like to blame perimenopause for all of our problems, but the hard truth is that stress is usually at the root of most problems. Cortisol is the "mean girl" in your body's neighborhood. She is completely disruptive when your stress is constant, partying at all hours of the day and night and keeping everyone else in the neighborhood jacked up and wonky as well.

The best way to test cortisol is at four points during the day with a saliva or urine test. Urine testing has an added advantage in that it allows the clinician to look at cortisol and its metabolites as well as cortisone, the inactive form of cortisol. The four-point diurnal test, also called a four-point cortisol curve or circadian cortisol pattern, reveals cortisol levels throughout the day and allows health care providers to pinpoint issues with the central stress response system.

Let's take a look at what is happening when the riot in your body due to stress is occurring.

Stress derails progesterone's work

First, cortisol can block your body's progesterone receptors. So you may have plenty of progesterone being made, but if cortisol is sitting in progesterone's seat, then progesterone can't do its job. I already mentioned that the body makes cortisol at the expense of all other hormones, and progesterone is used to make cortisol, so "cortisol steal" is also a possible reason for low progesterone.

Decreased sensitivity to estrogen

When cortisol is high in the brain, it is less sensitive to estrogen. Under normal circumstances, hot flashes are a symptom of estrogen deficiency. But sometimes, it's a signal that brain sensors have been altered by cortisol. That's why hot flashes can occur in women who have reasonable estrogen levels but are experiencing lots of stress. If estrogen is added with the intention of treating hot flashes in a woman whose estrogen levels are reasonable, the outcome will be weight gain in the hips, water retention, and mood swings—all signs of too much estrogen. And the hot flashes won't go away, either.

Thyroid hormone and cortisol depend on each other

One of cortisol's more important functions is to work with thyroid hormones at the cellular level. Cortisol makes thyroid hormones work more efficiently. A balanced amount of cortisol (not too high or low) is very important for normal thyroid function. This is why a lot of women who have a cortisol imbalance may also have low thyroid symptoms but still have normal results on a thyroid test.

Every cell in the body has receptors for both cortisol and thyroid hormones, and almost every process that goes on in cells requires the thyroid to be humming along at peak performance levels. Too much cortisol can create a problem of thyroid resistance where the tissues fail to respond to the hormone. This resistance can also be seen with other hormones such as insulin, progesterone, estrogen, testosterone, and even cortisol itself. Resistance means the body has to work harder and harder to make more of the other hormones when cortisol is high. The bottom line is that chronic stress makes you feel rotten because none of the hormones are allowed to function as they should.

Stress plus insulin equals overeating

Under stressful conditions, cortisol provides the body with glucose for energy by tapping into protein stores. However, high cortisol over the long-term results in too much glucose, which then leads to increased blood sugar levels. Over time, the pancreas, which produces insulin, struggles to keep up with the body's needs, and blood sugar remains high. The end result of this cycle is that cells are starved of energy because there's not enough insulin to help the glucose get into cells. When cells find themselves in this situation, they send out an SOS to the brain, which then sends out hunger signals. This is how stress leads to overeating and weight gain. Any unused glucose that is circulating is eventually stored as body fat.

DHEA protects against signs of aging

DHEA (dehydroepiandrosterone) is one of your male hormones (also known as androgens). The other male hormone is testosterone. In the hormone cascade, flexible DHEA turns into either testosterone or estrogen. In women, it is more likely to head down the testosterone route. In men, it's the opposite.

DHEA works to counter the effects of cortisol, and because of this, it is a very powerful anti-aging hormone. Since cortisol and DHEA have opposing effects, practitioners look at the ratio of the two to each other. When cortisol is disproportionately greater than DHEA, the ratio is high. This can result in the following:

- Increased inflammation
- Poor immune function
- Insulin resistance
- Compromised thyroid, pancreas, and ovarian function
- Inability to detoxify heavy metals
- Bone breakdown
- Poor memory

A lower than normal ratio indicates that something is amiss in the hypothalamic pituitary axis (HPA), leaving the body unable to respond well to stress.

What You Need to Know About "Adrenal Fatigue"

Adrenal fatigue is all over the internet and has become a popular diagnosis among patients and practitioners, at least within the functional and integrative medicine worlds. Symptoms include everything from fatigue, insomnia, and brain fog to things such as joint pain, allergies, and weight gain. If you search for adrenal fatigue online, you'll see usually a bullet point list of every symptom under the sun, so it's very nonspecific. The term "adrenal fatigue" implies that our adrenal glands are fragile and subject to wearing out. Nothing could be further from the truth. The adrenals are actually very powerful and are responsible for cranking out stress hormones our whole lives. Then, in perimenopause and menopause, they also begin to pick up the slack of hormone production after the ovaries go into retirement.

If you look online for information about adrenal fatigue, you'll find experts divided into two camps. One camp believes that it affects hundreds of millions of people around the world and may be at the root of most modern disease. The other camp does not share this belief. So the question is, does adrenal fatigue really exist?

There are two primary problems with the adrenal fatigue idea. First, most people with so-called "adrenal fatigue" don't have low cortisol levels. Remember, most of us are living high-stress lives and our bodies are cranking out plenty of cortisol—it may just not be in the active form that works on cells. When cortisol is low, it's rarely because the adrenals are pooped and unable to produce it. It's more likely that Mother Nature is putting the brakes on you to send a message.

Most people don't have low cortisol

Adrenal fatigue is best diagnosed by using a saliva cortisol or dried urine test. Cortisol that's measured in saliva is in the unbound or free form. This means it's not bound to a protein carrier in the bloodstream. This free portion is the most potent form of cortisol and is what does the job at receptors, but it only represents about 3-5 percent of the total cortisol in the body at any given time. The rest of the cortisol hangs around in inactive cortisone or is cleared by several metabolic pathways before it's excreted in the urine. It's more common when people have low free cortisol for them to have either normal or high total cortisol. As I mentioned earlier, dried urine (DUTCH) testing has the added benefit of measuring the various metabolites of cortisol, allowing the clinician to better target interventions.

When cortisol is low, it's rarely because the adrenals are tired and unable to produce it

It's more likely that the body has slowed down the stress response axis in order to make *you* slow down. When we're exposed to stress over a long period of time, our bodies have a feedback mechanism that they use to protect us from the effects of high cortisol by decreasing the sensitivity of some receptors that are involved. The body is trying to prevent harm to you, but unfortunately, that ends up leading to a decreased ability to produce cortisol in the face of future stress. This has to do with brain signals, however, and not the adrenals' ability to make cortisol.

Why understanding this matters

All of this talk about terminology is not just splitting hairs. If a woman is falsely diagnosed with "adrenal fatigue" because testing is done using the incorrect method or the timing of the test is off, there's a good chance that the management strategy may do more harm than good. Treatments such as hydrocortisone or licorice that raise cortisol could worsen the situation if used inappropriately. This is one reason I now use the DUTCH urine test to measure cortisol; it reports all of the metabolites as well as cortisone (the inactive form of cortisol) and gives a clearer picture of what's really going on with stress hormones.

The Problem with Numbing Behaviors as a Stress-Management "Strategy"

Let's be honest. Unhealthy food (sugar in particular) and wine are perimenopausal go-tos for many women. They take the edge off anxiety and overwhelm, give us a hit of dopamine and allow us to feel a sense of relief. And while numbing can seem like a good idea in the moment, there are hidden dangers lurking in this management strategy.   One in four people in our culture is taking prescription pain medicine, and the rate of addiction to food, cigarettes, alcohol, video games, texting, and personal electronics is growing rapidly. Addictive substances and behaviors achieve their effects by imitating or enhancing the functions of our neurotransmitters. We numb ourselves from the pain, frustration, and anxiety of our lives. But if our lives are so stressful and uncomfortable that we need to constantly numb ourselves, then perhaps we need to learn how to live more creatively, instead. Creative living can change our brains and bring a sense of calm and peaceful rhythm.

Alternatives to numbing behaviors

When you're tempted to zone out and hit the potato chips, your best first step is to identify what you're really feeling. Your brain may tell you that you need that third glass of wine, but trust me, you don't. Ask yourself what it is you really need in that moment. Maybe you're depressed or lonely. If so, call someone who cheers you up or give your dog or cat some love. Maybe you're anxious. Try having a dance party in your living room or taking a fast walk. Exhausted? Take a bath and go to bed. Bored? Read a book, get outside, or do something you really enjoy. The key here is to really get in touch with what you're feeling, and that can be very uncomfortable for many of us. We don't want to put ourselves under that kind of microscope. I get it, and I'm right there with you. But until you are aware of what's really going on, then numbing your feelings will be the order of the day.

Stress is a habit, just like brushing your teeth or hitting the snooze button. And like all bad habits that need to be broken, you need to create a new habit to replace it. It's not enough to go to a therapist once a week and then get pummeled by your life the other six days. Meditation or sitting quietly to get centered at the beginning of your day (no electronics allowed) will help calm your mind and set the right tone for the day ahead.

Lifestyle Solutions for Reducing Stress

There are many tried-and-true ways to reduce stress and maintain calm:

Turn "I can't" into "How can I?"

Many women believe they are at the mercy of whatever is going on around them. This is a limiting belief that can suck the life out of you if you don't spot it and create some boundaries. You are not in charge of solving everyone's problems. You are only in charge of solving yours. The next time you hear "I can't" coming out of your mouth, stop and flip that around. Ask yourself a high-quality question that begins with, "How can I…?" This, my Savvy Sisters, is guaranteed to change your stress level and your life. It is how solutions get found. You're welcome.

Exercise

Walk with a friend, join a yoga class, bike, or hike. Exercise is a great way to reduce stress and stay healthy. Schedule it on your calendar as a priority.

Talk

Share the things you're worrying about with a family member, BFF, or counselor. The best money I've ever spent was on therapy.

Eat well

Although eating chocolate may soothe stress in the short run, too much leads to its own set of problems. A healthier strategy is to eat three nutritious meals daily along with healthy snacks, including fresh fruits and vegetables.

Avoid caffeine and alcohol

Both can affect your cortisol levels. Caffeine is hard on your adrenals because it causes a cortisol spike followed by a quick crash depending on how well you metabolize caffeine. Herbal tea (iced, if hot flashes are an issue) provides a soothing alternative to caffeinated drinks. Although alcohol may make you feel relaxed and drowsy, it has actually been shown to interfere with sleep quality. And, as I've discussed before, the potential for abuse and other health risks makes it a poor option for stress reduction.

Sleep

Yes, I know. You'd sleep if you could! So make solving your sleep problems a priority. Maybe that means going on oral progesterone. Maybe it means logging off all screens after 5:00 p.m. Maybe it means getting your kids out of your bed. Maybe it means trying cognitive behavioral therapy. Whatever it takes, make it happen.

Add in pleasure

Pleasure means different things to different people. Treat yourself to a massage, manicure, or soothing bath. Enjoy a good book, music, a walk in the woods, or a favorite hobby. Find a creative outlet by enrolling in an art or music program. Volunteer for a cause you love. Make a list of ideas and post it somewhere you can see it.

Lighten up

Our lives are not meant to be heavy and hard. Joy is free and heals things medical science can't.

Practice gratitude

If joy isn't accessible to you just yet, start with a short gratitude practice every day. Take five minutes each day to focus on what you're grateful for. Be very specific so you can really get to the *feeling* each thing brings you. Get your mind focused on what is good and true.

Unplug regularly

We all need a break from electronics to reconnect with ourselves and those around us. Consider a short break (a day, a weekend) from electronics and social media. Put your cell phone out of sight or turn it off. If this idea causes you to hyperventilate, I'm definitely talking to Y.O.U. Trust me, you'll be fine.

Breathing techniques

Another effective stress-reduction method is to use deep-breathing exercises. Try this simple exercise and practice it often:

1. Sit in a straight-back chair with both feet on the floor.
2. Rest your hands on your abdomen.
3. Slowly count to four while inhaling through the nose and feel the abdomen rise.
4. Hold that breath four counts.
5. Then, slowly count to four while exhaling through the mouth—let the abdomen slowly fall.
6. Hold for four counts before inhaling again.
7. Repeat this exercise five to 10 times.

Guided imagery & meditation

If there's no extra time or money for a vacation, try a brief mental vacation using "guided imagery" to achieve a state of deep relaxation. Close your eyes and visualize a scene from your memory that brings joy. Allow your mind to get lost in that experience for a few minutes. Need more variety or have trouble summoning up an image? There are many apps available (often free) where you can download guided imagery sessions to use.

Herbal Supplements that Help Stress

Stress has affected people for thousands of years. In ancient times, people used herbal remedies found in traditional Chinese medicine and Ayurveda for relief. If you're skeptical, rest assured that more and more clinical studies are demonstrating the benefits of herbal medicines. Be sure to read Chapter 9 before picking out your own supplements. Here are some of my favorites.

Ashwagandha

Ashwagandha has a long history of use in traditional Ayurvedic medicine. The entire plant, from roots to seeds, has beneficial properties, especially when it comes to stress reduction. The benefits of ashwagandha are wide-ranging, but it's great for helping people to feel less stressed. One study from 2017 showed a 44 percent reduction in stress levels after taking ashwagandha, as opposed to just a 5.5 percent decrease in the group taking a placebo. A randomized 2012 clinical trial showed similarly impressive levels of stress reduction after just 60 days of use.

Rhodiola

Rhodiola is a plant native to the arctic regions of Asia and Europe. This plant, also known as Golden Root, is used for energy enhancement, to improve mood, and to reduce stress. In a 2009 double-blind study, rhodiola was shown to reduce stress and increase alertness in doctors on night shifts. The most extensively studied property of this herb is its ability to help people deal with fatigue. Since exhaustion often contributes to stress, anything that reduces fatigue can help in the battle against stress. Be aware that rhodiola can be energizing for some people, so do not take it late in the day.

Valerian root

Valerian root is well-known for helping with sleep issues, including insomnia. This is largely due to its calming, sedative effect. The best part? It doesn't have the unpleasant side effects of medications typically used for these symptoms, such as grogginess, nor does it lead to dependence. The worst part? It smells terrible. Lack of sleep makes dealing with stress much harder, so one of the best stress relievers is a good night's sleep. Valerian root may be a potent, low-risk tool in your de-stressing arsenal.

Bacopa monnieri

Bacopa monnieri is a perennial herb that has proven stress-reducing benefits. It's been used as part of Ayurvedic medicine for centuries to enhance learning, boost memory, sharpen focus, lower stress, and improve mood. Modern research has also focused on

B. monnieri's ability to relieve stress, which it achieves partly by lowering cortisol levels.

Vitamins and Minerals that Help Stress

Vitamin B complex

Stress depletes B vitamins. This is why B vitamins are so important. Choose a broad-spectrum product that does not contain folic acid. A significant proportion of the population is unable to convert folic acid to folate which can cause a buildup of it. Having too much folic acid in the body can result in side effects including digestive problems, nausea, loss of appetite, bloating, gas, a bitter or unpleasant taste in the mouth, sleep disturbances, depression, excessive excitement, irritability, and a zinc deficiency. More severe signs of folic acid toxicity include psychotic behavior, numbness or tingling, mouth pain, weakness, trouble concentrating, confusion, fatigue, and even seizures. Look for l-methylfolate or Quatrefolate to avoid the need for conversion from folic acid.

Magnesium

Magnesium is a mineral that is essential for muscle and nerve function. Multiple studies have shown that magnesium is especially crucial for sleep, and many a Savvy Sister in my practice (including me), has been helped by adding magnesium at bedtime.

These herbs and supplements are not the only alternatives to pharmaceuticals, but they are low-risk starting places for women who like a do-it-yourself approach. For more expert help, please feel free to schedule a consultation with me at: www.drannagarrett.com/lets-talk.

Chapter 9:
How to Safely Use the Supplements that May Be Helpful in Perimenopause

It's the middle of the afternoon, and you head to the fridge to grab your usual Diet Coke pick-me-up. If it weren't for caffeine, how would you get anything done? You know you'll pay for it tonight when you're tossing and turning, but whatever. A girl's gotta do what a girl's gotta do. No time for a nap.

Your energy level just hasn't been what it should be. Then you remember that one of your friends mentioned a supplement she's started taking that sounds too good to be true. So you hop in the car and head to Whole Foods. You're standing in the aisle and there's a whole smorgasbord of supplements staring back at you. And you can't for the life of you remember what the heck she said she was taking! So, you decide to create your own cocktail with a little of this and a little of that. And the next thing you know, you've dropped $200 without having the first clue about what you're doing or whether it's safe. Sound familiar?

Just Because You Can Doesn't Mean You Should

The supplement industry's market is as much as $37 billion a year, according to one estimate. Ads for these products can be found on internet pop-up windows, on social media, in magazine pages, and on TV. Supplements are sold in corner health stores, pharmacies, and big box grocery stores. But they don't come with explicit instructions on how much to take (only a suggested dose) or potential drug interactions, and this is where problems can arise.

Many of my clients prefer to go the "natural" route for balancing hormones. This generally means that they don't want to go on hormone replacement therapy—specifically, estrogen. Fortunately for me and my clients, there is a whole array of over-the-counter supplements out there that can be helpful. None of these products require a prescription, so they're super-convenient, but that doesn't mean they are always safe.

Here are two perfect examples of how problems can arise. One of my clients recently completed her salivary hormone analysis. When the results came back to me, her DHEA and testosterone levels were sky high. She is on a testosterone supplement, so that result was understandable. What didn't make sense was the DHEA level. She did not list it with her supplements, but I knew something was up. When I asked her about it, she mentioned she was taking 50 mg of DHEA daily. This dosage is widely available on the shelves of health food stores and on the internet, but experienced practitioners know the recommended dose for women is 5–10 mg/day. She was taking five times the recommended amount, and this is why her level was so high.

So what's the danger here? When DHEA enters the hormone cascade in the body, it is mostly likely to be converted to testosterone in women, thus adding to testosterone levels. Elevated testosterone causes irritability, acne, hair loss on the scalp (which my client was experiencing), and unwanted body hair growth among other things. There is also some evidence that it may increase cardiovascular health risks. Excess testosterone can also be converted to estrogen, thus contributing to estrogen dominance. This is an excellent example of how things can go horribly wrong if you don't know what you're doing.

Here's another example: someone posted in the Hormone Harmony Club that she had decided to try some over-the-counter estrogen cream her mother had been using. Believe it or not, estrogen cream is available on Amazon. It shocked me, too, when I first found it. This person was happily loading up on estrogen cream when I asked her if she'd had a hysterectomy. She replied no. Why is this a problem? Because unopposed stimulation of the uterine lining by the use of estrogen in women who still have a uterus can lead to uterine cancer. Again, a case of not having all the information before self-treating.

In my practice, supplements are second-line therapy to lifestyle changes. There is no way to supplement your way out of a poor diet, lack of sleep, lack of movement, unrelenting stress, or any other choices that you are making that your body doesn't like. If you've made positive changes and still aren't where you want to be, then it may be time to think about supplements. Before you spend your hard-earned dollars, however, do your research. Understand what you are trying to accomplish, and at the very least, ask your pharmacist for help. Manufacturers generally suggest "consulting with your physician." Save your breath because most MDs have no clue about supplements or drug interactions. Go straight to the pharmacist instead. (And if you're an MD who's reading this and you do know about supplements, my humblest apologies.)

How to source the best supplements

Before we get into specifics, let's talk quality. Over the last few years, there have been a number of stories in the news about supplements that were either contaminated or contained no active ingredients. These were generally sold through mass marketers. Quality matters. A lot. Herbs grown in China tend to be contaminated with heavy metals. Lower-quality supplements may contain fillers or undesirable dyes. Here are five simple things to look for that will help you in making your next dietary supplement purchase:

1. Choose additive-free supplements
Try to find a dietary supplement that is additive-free. This is important because many supplement manufacturers use fillers such as magnesium stearate and stearic acid during the manufacturing process. These additives help speed up the manufacturing process and production volume (i.e. profit), but they have absolutely no health benefits to you, and they are, in fact, potentially

harmful to both the immune system and the cardiovascular system. Try to find a brand that leaves out additives. Ask someone in the health food store/market to assist you, as they are typically aware of which products are additive-free and which are not. Also check for allergens such as soy, wheat, dyes, or genetically modified (GMO) ingredients. These can cause reactions if you are sensitive to them.

2. Choose a manufacturer that only uses the highest-quality ingredients

Choose a product whose manufacturer spares no expense in sourcing and testing the raw materials and ingredients for their product. The highest quality ingredients are usually sourced from the United States, Europe, and South America. A good manufacturer will test all of their ingredients in a laboratory for identity, strength, purity, and composition before they use them in their formulations. A product that simply says "pure" or "high quality" is not good enough without documented testing to back it up. I have a link to my "store" in the resources section. I carry and recommend only the highest quality brands such as Ortho Molecular, Thorne, Integrative Therapeutics, Pure Encapsulations, and Metagenics.

3. Search for a brand that is sold by the manufacturer

Did you know that many supplement companies do not make their own products? Many dietary supplements are actually produced and manufactured by a third party. It is worth it to search for a brand or product that is manufactured by the same company that is selling it to you. More importantly, look for a brand or product that is being produced in a GMP-certified (Good Manufacturing Practices) facility as outlined by the United States Food and Drug Administration. This process is governed by more than 140 standard operating procedures that are reviewed by the FDA with an actual site inspection of the manufacturing facility. The bottom line is, try to find a dietary supplement that has a manufacturer that controls every aspect of the quality of the product. A brand or product being sold to you by the same company that is manufacturing it will have a higher commitment to quality because their integrity is on the line.

4. Choose supplements that reveal the source of ingredients
Notice how the ingredients are listed in the "Supplement Facts" panel of the product, and look for information regarding the country where the product was grown. Avoid sources from Asian countries if possible.

5. Choose clearly targeted formulas
The best products on the market are brands that feature formulas designed to provide nutritional benefits with a clear focus. For example, a complete multivitamin that is specifically designed for men or for women is preferable because different genders have different nutritional needs. Condition-specific formulas help with specific problems such as stress, cardiovascular issues,

and joint pain. A superior brand or product will not make it complicated for you to understand what you are buying.

Nine Reasons Your Supplements May Not Be Working

If you're taking vitamin or herbal supplements and you're not getting the results you'd like, or your regimen seems to have stopped working, it may be time to take a deeper look at what's going on. There are two common misconceptions about natural remedies. First, there is no one single dietary change, supplement, treatment, or protocol that will "fix" a chronic health challenge. Second, natural remedies are what I call "root problem" remedies for health problems. The remedy itself doesn't do the work to fix the body, but rather it supports the entire function of the body to do what it does best—restore balance. Your body wants to stay in balance and it does everything it can to do exactly that. It's constantly scanning your landscape to detect, assess, and make a concentrated effort to restore homeostasis (balanced health). As long as you are giving it the building blocks for balance, it operates smoothly.

Before you get fed up and decide to toss your supplement regimen, let's take a look at nine of the reasons your results might be less than what you'd hoped for:

1. You haven't been on them long enough

I try to help my clients manage expectations when it comes to taking supplements, but occasionally I will have someone who is emailing me two days after starting something wondering why it's not working. Natural remedies generally take longer to work than pharmaceuticals, so you need to give your herbs and vitamins a good three-month trial at minimum.

2. You're not addressing underlying nutritional issues

You can't outrun a bad diet with handfuls of supplements. There is no substitute for good nutrition. This means eating adequate protein, not skipping meals, eating lots of fresh veggies, fruits and healthy fats, and drinking at least half an ounce of water or more per pound of body weight per day.

3. You're not managing stress

There are herbs and supplements that can help you achieve better balance for cortisol, but if you do not address your underlying stress there is no supplement that will "fix" this. It is easy to fall into the trap of believing that you are "stuck" with whatever life serves up. This limiting belief is a fast pass to burnout, exhaustion, and frustration—all of which take a toll on your adrenal health.

4. You have underlying hormone imbalances

You may have underlying sex hormone, cortisol, or thyroid imbalances that are preventing your supplements from working as well as they could. Testing can help identify these so they can be addressed and make your protocol more effective.

5. You have underlying gut health issues

Good health begins in your gut. If you have damage to the lining of your gut or issues with low stomach acid (the most common cause of GERD), then you may not be absorbing the nutrients from supplements into your body. Issues with constipation or diarrhea can also affect how supplements work.

6. You're buying poor-quality products

Buy your vitamins and herbs from a reputable supplier. As I mentioned before, many cheap store brands contain few or no active ingredients. Purchase brands that have been independently tested for quality. This is one situation where spending a little extra to get better brands is worth it.

7. Your protocol isn't the right one for you

It's easy to stand in the supplement aisle of the health food store and load up a basket of products. But how do you know what you need? Could you be making things worse by choosing the wrong herb? If you think your body needs a significant amount of support, it's worth paying an expert to help you. Get testing if needed, and let a professional create a management plan for you. Organic acid testing can be especially helpful when it comes to identifying nutrient deficiencies. (Organic acids are metabolic by-products of cellular metabolism and can be measured from a urine sample.)

8. You're taking an inadequate dosage

The recommended daily allowance (RDA) is just that. It's a recommendation for maintaining health, but not necessarily enough for healing. Often, that amount is not enough to do the job if you need extra support in some areas. An example of this is in the situation of low cortisol. Large doses of Vitamin C and B5 are needed to provide the building blocks for healing, yet the RDA for these two vitamins is much lower. Most vitamins are eliminated in urine if the body doesn't need them. The exceptions to this are Vitamins A, D, E, and K, which can be stored by the body, creating the possibility for toxicity from mega-doses.

9. Something in your life needs to change

If you're stuck in a soul-sucking job, your marriage is a mess, or your plate is ridiculously full of obligations, there is no amount of supplementation that will make it better. This is the time to re-evaluate every aspect of your life. Be the detective here…and be honest. It is much easier to stick to the surface things you're probably doing already (such as taking supplements) because it is much more comfortable to do this than to dig deep for what needs to be addressed. But ultimately, your healing depends on your willingness to get uncomfortable and do the real work that needs to be done.

Dr. Anna's Foundational Five Supplements for Hormone Harmony

Let's get down to the nitty-gritty. I don't believe anyone needs a suitcase full of supplements to feel their best. However, there are certain nutritional areas where we may come up short despite our best efforts. Here are my five most impactful choices for women who are going through perimenopause.

1. Magnesium

If you're a busy woman, chances are you're deficient in magnesium and don't even know it. This multitasking mineral is needed for your body to complete around 300 processes, many of which impact hormone balance, and it can be hard to get from food sources.

Signs of low magnesium

Low magnesium levels can cause:
- Muscle spasms that range from foot cramps to chest pain (always get chest pain checked out)
- Headaches

- Feeling constantly fatigued or weak
- Anxiety and edginess
- Loss of appetite
- Quick exhaustion during exercise: research has found that during moderate activity, women with low magnesium levels in their muscle are likely to use more energy and tire far more quickly.
- Insomnia: supplements are very effective for improving sleep quality and depth.

Magnesium can't be manufactured as a single molecule; it needs to be bound to something else to be stable, so the biggest difference in different magnesium products comes not from the magnesium itself (which is all the same) but from the molecule it's bonded to. The most common bonding agents are oxide, citrate, glycinate, taurate, sulfate, and threonate.

Magnesium itself is poorly absorbed (35 percent absorbed in the worst-case scenario and 45 percent absorbed in the best). Calcium and magnesium compete for absorption at doses higher than 250 mg, so if you take calcium and magnesium together, they will compete with each other (meaning you will absorb less of each). Also, high or low protein intake and phytates from some vegetables can reduce magnesium intake. Generally, if you're taking a magnesium supplement, it's best done on an empty stomach. Magnesium also absorbs well through the skin (potentially far better than through the digestive tract), so Epsom salt baths (magnesium sulfate) and magnesium lotions, gels, or oils (usually magnesium chloride) can be a great way to increase your body stores. Topical forms can be best if you're using magnesium for its muscle relaxation and calming properties. The recommended daily allowance (RDA) for magnesium is 120–400 mg of elemental magnesium.

The benefits and downfalls of different types of magnesium

Magnesium oxide

Magnesium oxide is simply bonded to oxygen, which is something your body needs, so there is nothing unnecessary in the product. This is the least absorbed form and the most likely to cause diarrhea. I don't recommend it. Most magnesium oxide products contain 140 mg.

Magnesium citrate

This is one of the most common forms of magnesium on the commercial market. This is magnesium bonded to citric acid, which increases the rate of absorption. This is the most commonly used form in laxative preparations. You are now warned! It is a good choice if you tend to be constipated. The dose is 160-320 mg daily.

Magnesium glycinate

This is my personal favorite and the one I use and generally recommend because it gets into the brain and is well absorbed from the GI tract. The glycine itself is a relaxing neurotransmitter and so enhances magnesium's natural relaxation properties. In my opinion, this is the best form for sleep. The dose is between 120 and 360 milligrams. Experiment to find what works best for you.

Magnesium taurate

This is a less common form and is typically taken for cardiac conditions and heart function in general. Magnesium helps the heart muscle relax and helps open blood vessels so more blood can be delivered to the heart tissue. Another benefit of taurine is that it turns into GABA, which, as I discussed earlier, helps with sleep and relaxation. The recommended dose is 400 mg at bedtime.

Magnesium sulfate and magnesium chloride

Both these forms are typically used topically, although there are some oral preparations available. Oral forms have a very strong laxative effect. Magnesium sulfate is best known as Epsom salts. When used in a bath or soak it is extremely relaxing to the muscles and can ease aches and pains. Epsom salt baths can also help to lower high blood pressure and reduce stress levels. Magnesium chloride is more common in the lotion, gel, and oil preparations, and it can be used topically for muscle cramps and relaxation.

Magnesium threonate

Magnesium threonate also crosses the blood-brain barrier and so has recently been studied for uses in Alzheimer's disease and other forms of cognitive decline. Additionally, it has the same benefits as any other magnesium, including enhancing sleep quality. The recommended dosage is 2,000 mg/day.

2. Chasteberry (Vitex agnus-castus)

Chasteberry has been used for centuries to help with menstrual problems such as PMS, irregular cycles, and low progesterone. There has been considerable research (mostly from Europe) suggesting the effectiveness of chasteberry in treating the symptoms of PMS, breast tenderness, and infertility related to elevated prolactin or low progesterone.

The therapeutic dose of chasteberry depends on the brand and the formulation you chose. Chasteberry is available in liquid, capsules, and tablets. Most clinical trials used a dose of 20–40 mg/day, although some have used doses as high as 1,800 mg/day. Problems associated with elevated prolactin may need higher doses.

Chasteberry is not associated with any serious side effects, but it can cause dizziness, abdominal cramping, nausea, fatigue, dry mouth, and skin reactions. It is also possible to see some changes in your period when you start taking chasteberry, but these tend to resolve over time. Because chasteberry can alter progesterone and possibly estrogen levels in your body, women with hormone-related conditions such as breast cancer should not use this supplement. It is also very important to understand that taking this herb may decrease the effectiveness of the combination hormonal contraceptives. **Taking chasteberry while using the oral contraceptive pill, the contraceptive patch, or Nuvaring for birth control increases the chance that you could get pregnant.**

3. Adaptogen blends

Adaptogenic herbs are safe, non-toxic herbs that support the adrenal glands, helping you respond to stress. They help regulate cortisol whether it's high or low and are one of my main go-to supplements for clients. Adaptogenic herbs can be found as single herbs in tinctures or capsules. Many can also be made into teas. Some of my favorites include: rhodiola, panax ginseng, ashwagandha, eleutherococcus, licorice root, tulsi (holy basil), maca, and reishi mushrooms. The choice of which herb to use depends on the symptoms you are experiencing, and I generally recommend blends of multiple adaptogens to my clients.

4. B-complex vitamins

The B vitamins, which include thiamine, niacin, B12, and folate are often referred to as the "stress" vitamins. There are many symptoms of B vitamin deficiency, and these include hair loss, tension, irritability, difficulty managing stress, poor concentration, and anxiety. B vitamins have a complex role in your body, and they are depleted by stress and some medications such as birth control pills. Ensuring you have optimum levels during perimenopause can help in a number of ways to support stress management.

5. Vitamin D with K2

Every cell in your body uses Vitamin D. Adequate intake is important for the regulation of calcium and phosphorus absorption as well as the maintenance of healthy bones and teeth. It has also been suggested that it may provide a protective effect against diseases such as cancer, type-1 diabetes, and multiple sclerosis.

The best way to get Vitamin D (which is actually a hormone) is by letting our skin convert sunlight to D3. Ten minutes of direct exposure without sunscreen is all you need daily. Even though that's a short amount of time, it can be challenging to schedule this, especially if you live in an area tends to be cloudy a lot or has short days in the winter. I supplement with a Vitamin D product that also contains Vitamin K2, which helps the D3 do its job. D3 and K2 work together to prevent calcium from depositing in the lining of the main arteries in your neck that feed blood to your brain. Calcification of these arteries can lead to heart disease and stroke. I generally recommend 5,000 IU of Vitamin D3 daily along with 100 mcg of Vitamin K2 to my clients, with a goal level of 50-70 ng/mL.

A note on progesterone therapy

You may wonder why progesterone cream is not on my Foundational Five list. The longer I practice, the more I believe that use of progesterone requires the guidance of an expert. Not everyone responds well to progesterone therapy, and if estrogen is not in the ideal range, it tends not to work. Also, low cortisol can lead to a negative response to progesterone. The only way to know whether these levels are where they need to be is to get tested. Testing is available direct-to-consumer, but some degree of expert interpretation is needed, especially for the DUTCH test, which is very complex.

We all want to feel and look our best. But it's important to approach supplementation safely. This means taking the time to understand what you're doing and how the different hormone pathways in the body work together. A DIY approach is not necessarily best. It's worth the investment to find a practitioner who can work with you to do testing for baseline hormone levels, create a plan for supplementation if needed, do follow up testing to make sure your goals are being achieved, and educate you. Taking matters into your own hands without knowing where you're starting from can be downright dangerous. Next time you're considering adding a supplement, don't assume it's safe. Make sure you do the research and talk to your pharmacist. Mention every single supplement that goes into your mouth or onto your skin. And remember, your doctor may not always be familiar with problems related to herbals and other supplements. You are your own best advocate, so do your homework.

Chapter 10:
How to Get the Care You Need (and Deserve) in Perimenopause

Lynn is experiencing many signs of perimenopause. She can't sleep, she's tired all the time, and she's anxious about everything. Her flooding periods have her homebound for three days of the month. Lynn went to her doctor and asked to have her hormones tested. He refused and told her that it wouldn't be useful because she was too young (42) and because hormone levels change constantly. He did do a folli- cle-stimulating hormone (FSH) test, and it was in "normal" range. She was offered birth control pills and an antidepressant, but she threw the prescrip- tions in the trash on her way out of the office. She knows there's something hormonal going on and desperately wants to get to the bottom of it. Lynn has tried everything she's read about with almost no suc- cess. She's frustrated and has no idea where to turn.

Being Your own Advocate

While there are many options for managing perimenopause on your own, the day may come where you have to enlist your doctor or other health care provider for more help. This, my Savvy Sisters, is where the rubber meets the road. This is where the knowledge and advocacy skills you've been acquiring up until now will pay off.

Here's what you're up against: most medical schools and residency programs don't teach aspiring physicians about menopause. Indeed, a recent survey reveals that just 20 percent of OB-GYN residency programs provide any kind of menopause training. Mostly, the courses are elective. And nearly 80 percent of medical residents admit that they feel "barely comfortable" discussing or treating menopause. This lack of knowledge also extends to practicing OB-GYNs. Many don't have sufficient knowledge about the nuances of menopause to offer their patients anything but the standard birth control pill or IUD option. A survey of more than 1,000 medical professionals (including doctors, physician assistants, and nurse practitioners) regarding their knowledge of hormone replacement therapy (HRT) for menopause symptoms showed that only 57 percent of physicians were up-to-date on their information. Suffice it to say, the picture isn't pretty.

In addition to a lack of training, there's another aspect to navigate. The United States medical system is set up such that your average physician has to see a patient every seven minutes if he or she wants to maintain the level of productivity that's required by many health systems. Productivity requirements have killed the doctor/patient relationship in many ways because who has the time to get to the bottom of an issue that can more easily be bandaged with an anti-depressant or birth control pills?

When I decided to create my business, I wanted to work with women who were looking for alternative solutions. That's where my expertise as a pharmacist comes in very handy. Many people think pharmacists only know about prescription drugs. *Au contraire*! In our six years of training, we are also taught about herbs, vitamins, and other natural alternatives. For me, this was the perfect marriage of my years of training and my desire to serve women who were like me. Not only am I passionate about helping women manage their perimenopause experience, I'm also fired up about teaching women how to advocate on their own behalf in a broken healthcare system.

As a pharmacist, I know I get treated differently by my doctor because I know what questions to ask and have already done my research. She knows that I know what I'm talking about. That's one of the perks of being in school forever. But what about the rest of the world? What about you? The good news is that you don't need a degree in healthcare to have an intelligent conversation about your needs and goals.

How do you develop confidence and muster the courage to find your voice and get your needs met? I've put together this list of scenarios with suggestions on how to handle them to help you start building confidence. The courage? Well, that just takes practice and requires a willingness to keep looking for answers. Your health depends on it. Let's look at some common situations you're likely to encounter as you navigate the healthcare system.

Your doctor tells you that what you're experiencing is all in your head

This makes my blood pressure go up just typing it. Above all else, trust that you know your body better than anyone. Never forget this. Even if your provider says, "It's all in your head," your body has innate wisdom that only you are aware of. Trust that wisdom and keep searching for the right caregiver until you find someone who is willing to listen and respect your point of view.

Your doctor dismisses you as being "too young" to be in perimenopause

Explain to your care provider that you've done some research, and you're aware that perimenopause can start as early as the mid-30s for some women. Have a written list of what you've been experiencing, and for extra credit, track your experiences through the month so your doctor can see if they follow a cyclical pattern. I cannot stress enough how helpful this is. Tell your doctor what you've done on your own to try to solve any problems and how well these approaches worked. Ask what kinds of testing might be available and whether he or she is willing to do the testing. Remember, your doctor has seven minutes for you, and the longer you are sitting there asking questions, the more likely they are to give you what you want just to get you out of there. The squeaky wheel gets the grease.

Your insurance won't pay for you to see a hormone specialist or an alternative provider

You need to ask yourself high-quality questions when it comes to your health. "Will my insurance pay for this?" isn't one of them. I get that finances can be a barrier, but money shouldn't be the only deciding factor. Higher quality questions might include:

- What is the return on my investment if I do XYZ? (It may not be financial.)
- How will feeling better impact my life?
- What's it costing me to do nothing?
- Do I really want my insurance company deciding how good I can feel?

Remember, instead of beginning your thought process with "I can't," begin with, "How can I...?" You are much more likely to land on a good solution if you approach what feels like an insurmountable barrier with a positive question.

You get into the exam room and feel flustered and rushed

When you meet with your provider, be organized and to the point. Think about what you want to talk about before your appointment and write your questions down in order of importance. If you need to, take a spouse or trusted friend with you to your appointment to be another set of ears. If your doctor is impatient or rushes you, start looking for another doctor.

You want to do research before your visit, but it all feels like a bottomless rabbit hole

OK, fair warning: it IS a bottomless rabbit hole. Do a little preliminary research about your symptoms, but not so much that you scare yourself to death. As you learned earlier, perimenopause has a 34-item (or more, depending on the source) laundry list of possible signs and symptoms, so you can't rely on anyone else's experience to look like your own. Know a little bit about what your options are and what you want for yourself. Here are some decisions you may need to make, so think about your preferences before you get in the exam room.

Are you willing to use hormones or not?

Research birth control pills, Mirena/Skylar IUDs, and bioidentical progesterone (oral and cream) so that you have an idea of side effects, dosing, and how each of these might affect what you're experiencing.

Are you willing to make big lifestyle changes or not?

Decide what your lines in the sand are. It could be the nightly glass of wine. Or chocolate. Maybe you're not planning to ever set foot in a gym. Let your provider know these things at the beginning of your conversation because if you don't buy into the plan, then it's pointless to pretend that you will. Be honest with yourself and your doctor.

Are you willing to take antidepressants or not?

Depending on what you tell your doctor about your symptoms, a prescription for antidepressants may be high on the list of things that will happen. In some cases, this is a perfectly appropriate step to take, especially if you are suicidal. But in other situations, it's a fast, easy (for the doctor) bandage to cover an underlying hormone imbalance that still won't be fixed. If this is a road you don't want to travel, say so.

Are you willing to take sleeping pills or not?

As I discussed in the sleep chapter, all sleeping pills carry a risk of dependence, and many women are not willing to take them because of that risk. The more clarity you have, the better able your provider will be to make helpful recommendations. And don't be afraid to say no if things are going in a direction you don't like. Remember, you are in charge, and a "doctor knows best" mindset will not serve you.

Your doctor is not helping, and you don't know where to turn

Consider working with an alternative provider. Most women wouldn't think about working with a Doctor of Pharmacy to get their hormones balanced. But I offer testing, customized management plans, and lots of hand holding. No, your insurance probably won't cover working with me, but what's it costing you to do nothing? Plus, I'll give you a level of care that you can't possibly get in a seven-minute visit. Other helpful alternative care providers include acupuncturists (great for hot flashes), massage therapists, naturopaths, and herbalists.

You downplay any symptoms or physical complaints you have when you're in the doctor's office

Many of the women that I talk to don't want to appear too needy or whiny, and so they downplay their level of suffering at their doctor's visit or they fail to mention major problems they're having. A Savvy Sister knows better. This is the time to speak up.

If you're embarrassed by whatever is going on, trust me, most providers have seen and heard it all if they've been in practice for more than a minute. The bottom line is that your doctor won't be able to help you if you aren't honest about what's happening and don't clearly and honestly present any physical or emotional complaints to her. Do her and yourself a favor by speaking up. This is where summoning your courage is important. A confident patient/client who is upfront about what's going on will get the best care.

Be sure you understand the doctor's answers, and don't be afraid to ask for further explanation

Just because your doctor thinks she's answered your questions doesn't necessarily mean she has. If your doctor explains something to you, but you're still unclear about it, ask for further explanation. Don't go home and wonder (or call later and get stuck in phone tree hell). Asking follow-up questions saves time for you and the doctor. Get information in writing and take notes if needed. People remember less than half of what is told to them in a doctor's visit, and with the menopausal crowd, it's probably less than that. I speak from experience.

If you're confused, ask for information in people-speak, not medical jargon. Often a doctor will tell you about procedures or treatments using technical language that you can't make heads or tails of. If you don't understand what is being said, you can't make educated decisions, which, in the long run, may not serve you well.

Once you and your provider have decided on a course of action, keep up your end of the deal

There are few things more frustrating from my standpoint as a care provider than creating an elegant management plan for my client only to have them do nothing. If you know deep down that you can't or won't adhere to the plan, don't say you will. Be honest. If you can't afford the medications that are recommended, let your doctor know. If the plan has too many steps and you just want the first one, ask for that. And then follow through on it.

You want to break up with your doctor

Your health care provider is in practice because she wants you to rock your mojo! Good communication skills are an important piece of this. But let's face it, sometimes it's just not a good fit and it's time to break up. The least mature way to leave your doctor is the sneak attack. This is when you sign a medical records release form and skedaddle with no explanation. A more grown-up way (which increases confidence and courage) is to talk to your doctor about why you're not clicking. Don't just run away and leave, because maybe something can be salvaged if you talk openly and honestly.

Your doctor refuses to test your hormones and tells you it's not worth doing

There is a great deal of confusing and conflicting information online and in the medical community when it comes to navigating perimenopause, and the controversy over hormone testing is no exception. Let's think of navigating hormone balance in terms of travel. I want to describe two scenarios for you. The first is a road trip. I'm sure you can picture it: suitcases packed, convertible top down, sunglasses on, your BFF riding shotgun beside you. The question is: do you need a map?

For some women, the answer might be no. They aren't on a specific timeline, they don't have a specific destination in mind, they will fuel up when they need to, and they'll eat or pull over to the side of the road and when the mood strikes. Some things might go well. Some things might not go well. They are kind of half-prepared for either. Basically, they have decided to wing the entire trip without a roadmap. For other women, that type of journey isn't their cup of tea. They have a specific timeline and a specific set of sights they want to see. These BFFs want a plan mapped out for them that will show them where they started, what they can expect along the route, and when they will arrive at their destination. They'll be able to look back and appreciate how far they've come.

When it comes to managing hormones, testing is one tool that a healthcare professional has in their toolkit that helps provide a roadmap. Testing is intended to be used in combination with conversations with the patient, as well as in consideration of other health conditions and the symptoms that are the most concerning. Healthcare professionals like to use testing to validate a certain set of assumptions ("I think she has estrogen dominance"), or question/rule out other possibilities ("I'm not sure if her depression and inability to concentrate are related to fluctuations in progesterone or a thyroid condition"). Testing can also be beneficial in determining a baseline for a woman, so that she knows what "normal" looks like for her. If the woman then introduces a new protocol, such as supplementation and/or hormone therapy, she and her health care professional will be able to look back to her baseline test to monitor and track results.

My second scenario is travel-related, too. We can all imagine that feeling of driving along in your car and glancing down at the dashboard only to realize your "check engine" light is on. Thoughts bounce around in your mind, ranging from "OMG, it's serious" to "I'm sure it's nothing." What do you do? Let's assume you drive straight to your local mechanic's shop to explain to him that your engine light has just come on and it's a concern for you. He has two options. He can put some duct tape over the light, or he can lift the hood and investigate and fix the root cause. Both options get rid of the light on your dash. Which do you prefer?

When a woman is experiencing hormone fluctuations in perimenopause, she may symptoms that are mildly noticeable or moderately inconvenient, or that are severe and disruptive to her quality of life (as they can be for approximately 20 percent of women). Symptoms are not a foregone conclusion for women in perimenopause; they are communication tools. Symptoms are your body's way of alerting you that something is off, something requires your attention, or that something may need a gentle tweak or a course correction. Rather than masking the symptom with duct tape, you're more likely to have a better health outcome if you look under the hood for the root cause and treating whatever you find. Hormone testing helps care providers confirm their hypothesis and uncover any underlying root causes.

It is true that hormone testing is a snapshot in time (as are all lab tests) and that levels fluctuate, but in my practice, I find testing useful (if done at the correct time in a cycle) for looking at the magnitude of the imbalances that may be present and the metabolic pathways the woman's body prefers. Yes, your estrogen may fluctuate, but if it's way out of balance with progesterone, that imbalance is unlikely to correct itself at certain times during the day or month.

Is testing necessary? I say yes, but with certain caveats. Do you like to travel without a map? If your answer is no, then perhaps you and your health care provider should discuss the possibility of testing. Finances might be a potential barrier to this. In the U.S., the cost for testing hormones will vary depending on your insurance coverage. If you are working with a naturopath or other non-physician health care professional, you will likely be paying for the hormone testing out of pocket. I hear many successful stories now of integrated health teams working together on solutions that are best for the patient. For example, if you're working with me, I may request tests that you can ask your family doctor for without the out-of-pocket expense. Not all doctors are willing to work in a collaborative way, but it is certainly better for the patient. So, my preference is a "test don't guess" approach. Having data allows me to create a plan that is customized to a client's specific needs, and to work with her doctor to get bioidentical hormones onboard if necessary.

The "test don't guess" approach is far superior to one of "guess and treat." Unfortunately, the latter approach still wins the day in clinical practice. Most physicians would never prescribe blood pressure drugs or cholesterol-lowering medication without monitoring the patient appropriately. Many, however, are willing to prescribe hormones without clearly understanding how the woman's body is using them. This can result in preventable adverse effects and poor clinical outcomes—not to mention unhappy patients.

Types of testing

There are three main types of tests: saliva, blood, and urine or dried urine.

Saliva testing gives free hormone levels, is noninvasive, is great for tests that require multiple collections, and has been the preferred method of many naturopaths and alternative health care providers. It's efficient because collection can be done at home with minimal instructions, no freezing or refrigeration is required, and samples are stable at room temperature for thirty days. Saliva testing is effective for monitoring hormone therapy that is administered orally, vaginally, or via pellets, as well as for determining cortisol levels for adrenal stress assessment. It is not effective for monitoring topical therapy.

Blood tests are commonly used by physicians and are considered the ideal method for measuring molecular structures too large to capture in saliva. (i.e. blood lipids, vitamin D and thyroid hormones). Blood testing is a broadly accepted method for measuring hormone levels, but it is not effective for monitoring topical or vaginal hormone therapy.

Dried urine testing is my preferred testing method. It provides the best way to measure hormone byproducts and provides the only gauge for measuring how the body is metabolizing its hormones. Dried urine testing allows for discreet, at-home collection of four to five samples, and it eliminates the disadvantages of the hourly urine collections that were necessary for the previous 24-hour urine testing versions. It is suitable for measuring hormone levels, determines cortisol production at four time points for stress assessment, and accesses melatonin production. It is not suitable for the ongoing monitoring of topical progesterone or vaginal hormone therapy.

Which hormones should be tested

If you're considering any testing, here are important tests to include:

DHEA sulfate

DHEA-S is a hormone that converts into other hormones, including estrogen and testosterone. DHEA contributes to optimal adrenal function and your feeling of overall well-being. The ratio of DHEA-S to cortisol can give information about stress-related effects on adrenal function.

Estradiol

Estradiol is the main type of estrogen produced in the body, secreted by the ovaries and to a lesser extent in the adrenals. The balance of estrogen to progesterone is vital to hormone health.

Testosterone

In women, the ovaries' production of testosterone maintains a healthy libido, strong bones, muscle mass, and mental stability.

Progesterone

Progesterone is a hormone that stimulates the uterus and prepares it for pregnancy. It also regulates the menstrual cycle. As I mentioned previously, low levels of progesterone can cause insomnia, irritability, anxiety, and heart palpitations (among other things). Ideally, this test should be done between day 19–21 of your cycle (if still regular).

Thyroid

This includes checking your TSH (thyroid-stimulating hormone), free T3, free T4, and thyroid antibodies. Symptoms of perimenopause and a thyroid disorder can be very similar. This is best checked by blood tests.

Cortisol

Cortisol is a stress hormone, and high or low levels can throw your whole hormone symphony out of tune. The gold standards for testing are saliva at four or more points during the day or the DUTCH test which measures cortisol and cortisone (the inactive form of cortisol) as well as the metabolites of both.

The bottom line on testing

I speak with so many women who are frustrated when their doctors don't see the value in testing hormone levels. It's a common story. And it's important for women to understand the following:

Getting a follicle-stimulating hormone test for menopause is unnecessary

Unless you are in your 20s or 30s, there's almost never a good reason to test FSH. This test is used to determine how close you may be to menopause. But it fluctuates from month to month and tells you nothing about hormone imbalances. If you're in your 40s or 50s and you're experiencing any of what I've talked about so far in this book, and still having periods (occasional or regular) you are 99.9 percent likely to be in perimenopause. If you've had a period in the last 12 months, you are not in menopause.

Testing is not always a prerequisite for treatment

Every woman is different. And so is every health care professional. Some doctors feel confident prescribing hormone therapy or a new health regimen to certain patients who present with classic symptoms. For example, if a woman's chief complaint is vaginal dryness, she doesn't need a hormone test to confirm it—she needs treatment.

Hormone testing is a snapshot in time

Our hormones—especially in perimenopause—are fluctuating all the time. They vary from month-to-month, week-to-week, day-to-day, and even hour-to-hour. You could test in the morning and again at night and produce different results. For this reason, hormone testing is considered a guide—a support rather than the definitive be-all answer to your concerns. A trained clinician will look at your lab results for patterns, analyze the magnitude of any hormone imbalances, and use your history to make decisions.

There are a variety of ways to request hormone testing.

As I mentioned, testing hormone levels is only one tool that your health professional has for helping to guide you and recommend the best protocol for you and your particular situation. Your doctor might not be trained in hormone balance and may be hesitant to do testing because he or she isn't sure what to do with the results. If you've determined that hormone testing might be beneficial for you, and you've asked your doctor but have been met with some resistance, consider the following approaches (adapted from Dr. Sara Gottfried's The *Hormone Cure*):

- "I just read a book on perimenopause and because I'm experiencing [insert your symptoms], I'm wondering if you'd be willing to order a blood test for me?"
- "I've read there is a possible link between [fill in your particular experience] and [hormone name]. I'm interested in pursuing testing, so I can get past this and get on with enjoying midlife."
- "I understand you may not see the value in testing, but I love data and tracking my own

health. Is there someone you can refer me to who'd be willing to order the tests?"
- Do not demand anything. Doctors are human beings and appreciate being treated as such. If you can't get the help you're seeking, move on to another provider.

If the information above made your eyes glaze over, thank you for jumping to these final paragraphs. I believe it's important for you to have this information on hormone testing, so you can have more informed, productive, and engaged conversations with your health team. Are you expected to know what tests to order, or what method of collection would be best, or what the numbers mean on your lab results? Absolutely not. That's a job for someone like me.

Are you expected to be the captain of your own midlife team? One hundred percent! In order to be proactive and advocate for your own health, you do need to understand the context of the conversation and what your options are. Know this: there is no hormone test that can tell you or your doctor what treatment protocol or dosage is right for you. Hormone balance is very individual, and tests, as we've discussed, are merely a guide. I always recommend you work with an experienced professional who can not only request and interpret your test results, but who can also recommend nutritional and lifestyle options—with or without the inclusion of hormone therapy.

Chapter 11:
Hysterectomy 101: What You Need to Know Before Surgery

Here's a note I got from a woman in the Hormone Harmony Club who was desperately seeking help after her hysterectomy.

"Surgical menopause is kicking my butt! Two years ago, I had my uterus removed due to fibroid issues. At that time my ovaries were great; no issues. I started having some pain a few months after surgery. I finally went in and learned I had a five-inch-long tumor connected to my right ovary and bad endometriosis (which I'd never had before). My doctor took both ovaries, fallopian tubes and my appendix to top it off. I had no idea these symptoms would be so rough. I opted not to take estrogen as I assumed I could handle this. My doctor told me it was my choice. I am 40 years old and in full blown menopause. Hot flashes and night sweats are the worst. But I've also noticed weight gain, heart palpitations and sore joints. I am now considering taking estrogen. I am six weeks into this and just not sure what to

do. I am nervous and tired of dealing with all of this."

Why we Need to Talk About Hysterectomies

You may wonder why there's a chapter on hysterectomy in a book about perimenopause. It's because there's a good chance it may happen to many women before they get to menopause. About 55 percent of hysterectomies are performed on women between the ages of 35 and 49.

Women living in the southern U.S. experience the highest rate of hysterectomy, followed by those living in the Midwest. Those living in the west have the lowest, with a rate about two-thirds that of southern women. Southern women are also more likely to be younger when they have a hysterectomy, with the average age being 41.6, while women in the northeast are the oldest, with an average age of 47.7 when undergoing the procedure.

There's a tendency on the part of some gynecologists to look at the uterus and ovaries as "spare parts" once the patient has had her children. And for the unsuspecting woman who doesn't know better, removal of everything may seem like a good idea. That is a line of thinking that needs to change. A hysterectomy can be life-changing in good and bad ways. For the woman who's been battling her uterus and its antics all her life, it may be the best treatment option. But the flip side is instant menopause for those who choose to, or must, have their ovaries removed along with the uterus. This is not a decision that should be made lightly, and my hope in giving you this information is that you will know more about what's to come and thoroughly think through your decision should you be faced with having to make the choice. Let's dig in.

Types of Hysterectomy

All hysterectomies include removal of the uterus, but the type of procedure used often depends on the condition being treated. Your doctor will make a recommendation for the type you need. I am not a surgeon, nor am I qualified to speak about details of these procedures, so I am including quite a bit of detail from the Health Communities website here (see references) so that you'll know the options available and be able to ask questions. A hysterectomy is not just removal of parts that are contributing to your problems It can have far-reaching implications for your overall health, and you need to be able to advocate for yourself.

Partial or supracervical hysterectomies

In a partial or supracervical hysterectomy, the upper portion of the uterus is removed, leaving the cervix intact. Improved sexual function has often been cited as one of the primary reasons not to remove the cervix at the time of a hysterectomy, but multiple studies have shown no clear benefit to sexual satisfaction from either removal or preservation of the cervix. These studies looked at several factors, such as sensation during intercourse, ability to achieve orgasm, and pain with intercourse; a supracervical hysterectomy was not shown to be any better than a total hysterectomy when it came to these factors.

Pelvic organ prolapse is a condition where the uterus, bladder, or intestines may create a bulge in the vagina (patients are often told that their "organs have dropped"). One proposed benefit of leaving the cervix in place after a hysterectomy is to reduce the risk of this happening. Again, research has demonstrated this to be untrue; removing the cervix does not predispose patients to a higher risk of prolapse.

Complete or total hysterectomies

A complete or total hysterectomy involves the removal of both the uterus and the cervix. This is the most common type of hysterectomy performed. Hysterectomy with bilateral salpingo-oophorectomy (BSO) is the removal of the uterus, cervix, fallopian tubes, and ovaries. Radical hysterectomy is an extensive surgical procedure in which the uterus, cervix, ovaries, fallopian tubes, upper vagina, some surrounding tissue, and lymph nodes are removed. The choice of which to use depends on the condition being treated and the preferences of the woman. A radical hysterectomy is less common than BSO and is typically used for a diagnosis of cancer.

Surgical techniques for hysterectomy

Traditionally, hysterectomies have been performed using a technique known as total abdominal hysterectomy (TAH). However, in recent years, two less-invasive procedures have been developed: vaginal hysterectomy and laparoscopic hysterectomy.

In a total abdominal hysterectomy, the surgeon makes an incision approximately five inches long in the abdominal wall, cutting through skin and connective tissue to reach the uterus. The cut can be either vertical (running from just below the navel to just above the pubic bone), or horizontal (running across the top of the public bone). This is also known as a bikini-line incision.

One advantage of total abdominal hysterectomy is that the surgeon can get a complete, unobstructed look at the uterus and surrounding area. There is also more room in which to perform the procedure. This type of surgery is especially useful if there are large fibroids or if cancer is suspected. Disadvantages include more pain and a longer recovery time than other procedures, as well as a larger scar.

A vaginal hysterectomy is done through a small incision at the top of the vagina. The uterus (and cervix, if necessary) is separated from its connecting tissue and blood supply and removed via the vagina through this incision. If the cervix is not being removed, the incision is made around it, and it is reattached when the surgery is finished. This procedure is often used for conditions such as uterine prolapse. Vaginal hysterectomy heals faster than abdominal hysterectomy, results in less pain, and generally does not cause external scarring unless laparoscopic assistance is used.

In a laparoscopic hysterectomy, special surgical tools are used to operate through small incisions in the abdomen and vagina. There are two types of laparoscopic hysterectomy: laparoscopically assisted vaginal hysterectomy (LAVH) and laparoscopic supracervical hysterectomy (LSH). LAVH is similar to vaginal hysterectomy, in which the uterus and cervix are removed through an incision at the top of the vagina; however, the surgeon also uses a laparoscope (miniature camera) inserted into the abdomen to see the uterus and surrounding organs. Other laparoscopic tools are inserted into abdominal incisions to detach the uterus before removing it. LSH is performed entirely through small abdominal incisions, using laparoscopic tools to remove just the uterus. Since the cervix is not removed, the uterus is detached and removed in small pieces through the incisions. No incision is made at the top of the vagina.

Both types of laparoscopic hysterectomy cause less pain and have faster recovery times than TAH and produce minimal scarring. Laparoscopic surgery is used about 45 percent of the time now for hysterectomy. However, not all gynecologic surgeons offer it. If your doctor suggests that you are not a candidate for this type of surgery, ask, "Do you do a lot of minimally invasive surgery?" If they don't, it could be they are not up on the latest surgical techniques, and you may want to seek a second opinion.

Even though hysterectomy is the second-most common surgery for women in the United States, myths about removal of the uterus abound. If you are about to have this surgery, a heart-to-heart discussion with your gynecologist is essential. If your doctor is recommending a hysterectomy, there are several things (in addition to the type of surgery) you'll want to consider before going ahead. Here are important questions you need to ask and understand the answers to.

Can I avoid a hysterectomy?

Depending on the condition you are dealing with, you may be able to keep your uterus intact. Alternatives exist for about 90 percent of hysterectomies that surgeons do. Fibroids, for example, may be treated using a nonsurgical procedure called uterine artery embolization that cuts off a fibroid's blood supply. Another option to treat fibroids is myomectomy, which removes fibroids but spares the uterus. For heavy bleeding, an ablation procedure, which freezes or burns the uterine lining, may be a treatment option. For adenomyosis, a condition that occurs when the tissue that normally lines the uterus (endometrial tissue) grows into the muscular wall of the uterus, birth control pills and NSAIDs may be enough to control symptoms.

Will a hysterectomy CURE my problem?

Removal of your uterus and/or ovaries is major surgery and has long-lasting implications for your health. Unfortunately, it can be the path of least resistance for some doctors.

Examples of when surgery may not be the cure include situations such as endometriosis, where there is a possibility that the endometrial tissue will regrow in the abdominal cavity and cause problems outside of the uterus. In fact, endometriosis, a condition marked by severe menstrual cramps, chronic pain, and painful intercourse, is not cured by removal of the uterus, according to the Office on Women's Health at the U.S. Department of Health and Human Services. Of the many treatment options, which include pain medications and hormone therapies, hysterectomy with removal of the ovaries is not a first-line treatment for endometriosis.

A hysterectomy may also be recommended for depression, but unless the ovaries are removed, it is unlikely to fix the underlying depression, which is most likely due to hormone imbalance. Your uterus itself does not cause depression. In younger women who have cycle-related persistent depression as well as other cyclical problems of bleeding, pain, and headaches, hysterectomy with removal of the ovaries (bilateral oophorectomy) will usually cure these problems. However, the "instant menopause" this creates sets up issues with bone health and cardiovascular risk unless hormone replacement therapy (HRT) is used.

While removal of the uterus may be avoided in many of the situations above, it could be a real medical necessity if you have invasive cancer of the reproductive organs such as the uterus, cervix, vagina, fallopian tubes, or ovaries.

Can I keep my ovaries?

During surgery, your doctor may remove one or both ovaries and your fallopian tubes as well as your uterus. Ovaries are where estrogen, progesterone, and the male hormone testosterone are produced. These are all critical for sexual health, cardiovascular health, and bone health. Losing both ovaries means these hormone levels drop overnight. This is extremely hard on your body and can result in a sudden, wide array of menopause symptoms for most women. If you can keep your ovaries, do it, but be aware that the blood supply can be disrupted during surgery, which may cause damage and failure three or four years after surgery. That timespan, however, may be enough for you to naturally enter menopause.

Will I go into menopause right away?

Many women expect to start having crazy hot flashes, mood swings, and night sweats all the time after a hysterectomy, but this is a myth. You won't have periods after your uterus is removed, and you can't get pregnant, but that doesn't necessarily mean you go into menopause right away. The only women who have "instant menopause" are those who aren't already in menopause and who have ovary removal during the procedure.

If surgery is limited to the uterus, you will likely have a few good years of hormone production. As I mentioned above, there's a chance the surgery itself may cause the ovaries to lose function after a few years because of a disruption in blood supply, but a few lucky ladies sail on to complete their journey with few symptoms.

Do I need hormone replacement therapy?

This is a conversation that definitely needs to happen before surgery if you are having a total hysterectomy, especially if you are younger than the typical menopause age of 51. As I mentioned previously, a total hysterectomy puts you into menopause overnight, which is tremendously hard on the body. You do not want to be facing a hormonal nightmare after surgery. Most women feel better using a combination of estrogen and progesterone—with or without testosterone—since these hormones are depleted after removal of the ovaries.

Some doctors still subscribe to old-school thinking and may tell you that you don't need progesterone since you no longer have a uterus to protect from the effects of estrogen. Do not accept this short-sighted point of view. Many doctors don't understand the difference between synthetic progestins and bioidentical progesterone. Synthetic progestins are chemical compounds that are somewhat similar to what your body makes naturally, but they have been altered enough that they can be patented and sold by drug companies. Bioidentical progesterone is exactly the same compound your body makes, and for that reason, it cannot be patented and sold for huge profits. This is a situation where it is important to advocate for yourself. Bioidentical progesterone has positive effects on the body that go far beyond uterine protection. These include helping with anxiety and mood swings, bone health, nerve health, and weight management. Request that you be prescribed bioidentical estrogen (estradiol) in a topical form (patch, spray, cream, or gel) along with progesterone capsules or cream. Progesterone cream is available over-the-counter or by prescription. If you try this combo and still aren't feeling your best, ask to try testosterone. Testosterone must be compounded by a pharmacy since no products are commercially available for women. It can come in the form of topical cream or pellets that are inserted under the skin for slow release. These approaches are not appropriate for women who have or have had estrogen-fed cancers unless an oncologist gives the OK.

How soon can I have sex after surgery?

The answer to this really depends on the type of hysterectomy: partial, total, or radical. As a reminder, a partial hysterectomy involves removing your uterus but preserving your ovaries, a total hysterectomy removes your uterus and ovaries, and a radical hysterectomy involves removing the uterus, ovaries and cervix. Waiting two to four weeks to get back to sex is generally OK, with your doctor's go-ahead, if your cervix was not removed along with your uterus. But if your cervix was removed, it takes about six weeks for the back of the vagina to heal.

Be sure to be specific about what you mean by "sex." Are you asking about vaginal intercourse? Orgasm, oral sex, and vibrator use without penetration may be fine, but your questions need to be clear.

How much recovery time should I expect?

Depending on the procedure, you may have a brief recovery time in the hospital, or you may go home the same day. Your recovery time at home will vary, again depending on the procedure you had. Heavy lifting will not be allowed for all types of procedures.

Abdominal hysterectomy

Most women go home two or three days after this surgery, but complete recovery takes from six to eight weeks. During this time, you need to rest at home. You should not be doing housework or exercise until you talk with your doctor about restrictions. There should be no lifting for the first two weeks. After 6 weeks, you can begin getting back to your regular activities.

Vaginal or laparoscopic assisted vaginal hysterectomy (LAVH)

A vaginal hysterectomy is less surgically invasive than an abdominal procedure, and recovery can be as short as two weeks. Most women go home either the same day or the next. Walking is encouraged, but not heavy lifting.

Laparoscopic supracervical hysterectomy (LSH)

This procedure is the least invasive and has a fairly short recovery period (1-2 weeks).

What can I expect psychologically after surgery?

Many women are nothing but delighted to never have to deal with the issues that caused them to have a hysterectomy in the first place: no more flooding periods, and no more pain from fibroids. For some women, a hysterectomy is life-saving. But there's another side to having this procedure done. For some women, the emotional trauma of hysterectomy may take much longer to heal than the physical effects. Feeling grief or having a sense of loss after a surgery is normal, but many women struggle with feeling less feminine since they can no longer have children or periods.

Your likelihood of experiencing psychological and emotional problems after the hysterectomy appear to be related to whether you suffered from such problems before the surgery. If you faced depression or anxiety before the surgery, you have a higher risk of facing them after surgery. Many women in midlife face major career and family changes. A hysterectomy, especially one that results in menopause, may exacerbate that stress. Be on the lookout for postoperative depression and get professional help if you need it.

A hysterectomy is major surgery and has health implications far beyond the actual removal of the uterus, especially if your ovaries are removed too. As I mentioned earlier, ovary removal creates "instant menopause" and all the symptoms that go along with it. Even if you keep your ovaries, there can still be health risks. A recent study showed that women who kept their ovaries are still at higher risk for high blood pressure, obesity, and coronary artery disease. Ovary retention also means it's possible to still get ovarian cancer. Unless you ask, certain critical and highly sensitive topics might not come up when you discuss hysterectomy pros and cons with your doctor. So speak up and get specific. Find out what a hysterectomy could mean for your sex life, your hormones, and your future before you have the surgery.

Chapter 12:
What Comes Next?

Congratulations! You are now officially a Savvy Sister (provided that you didn't just jump to the end of the book). I spent a lot of time thinking about what I wanted to leave you with at the end of this. I think there are two things I want you to walk away with. First, there is hope. As with any other season of your life, perimenopause is what you make of it. Second, suffering during this time of your life is optional. I have given you the tools you need to begin making a big difference in how you feel, or (if you haven't reached perimenopause yet) to begin planning for how you'll approach it.

One of the questions I am asked on a regular basis is, "Will this getter better when I reach menopause?" And the answer is, it depends. For many women, the fall of hormones to post-menopausal levels is what they need to feel as if a new normal has arrived. For others, estrogen dominance symptoms continue because of ongoing hormone imbalances related to lifestyle, stress, and exposure to xenoestrogens. And for a third group, different symptoms arise, such as vaginal dryness and hot flashes. What you experience is largely related to genetics, hormone balance, and the lifestyle choices you make.

If you're just starting the process of perimenopause, you have a big advantage over your sisters who are nearing the end of it. You have time to really consider what you want for your long-term health and an opportunity to take the perimenopause bull by the horns. You've read a lot of information here, and now it's time to put together your Hormone Harmony Action Plan for success. Today is a perfect time to start! If you're still not 100 percent sure whether you're in perimenopause or not, you can find out by taking my quiz at: www.perimenopausequiz.com.

The Power of a Positive Mindset

Step one in your Hormone Harmony Action Plan is creating a powerful mindset. I cannot say enough about this. This is the habit that helps create the most success. Positive thinking won't create success on its own, but it certainly goes a long way to motivate you to take action. I learned this when I quit smoking. When I allowed myself to get caught up in negativity, I failed. But when I learned how to squash negative thoughts and flip them to better-feeling ones instead, I succeeded. Start by becoming more aware of your negative self-talk. I have my clients track this during the day. Keep a little tally sheet, noting each time you have a negative thought. Soon you'll recognize patterns and situations that bring about negative thinking.

If you fear perimenopause and menopause and you are hyper-focused on every twinge and hangnail, you will definitely have a rough ride. Think back to puberty. Did you spend all of your time obsessing about your body and what was going on? Of course not. And this transition is really no different. It's just the other end of the reproductive spectrum. As I mentioned earlier in the book, every thought is a choice. But choosing better thoughts takes practice. Two books I highly recommend for help in beginning a mindset/thought work practice are *Loving What Is* by Byron Katie and *Self-Coaching 101* by Brooke Castillo. Both books offer clear processes to work through to flip negative thinking. Byron Katie also has videos on her website (http://www.thework.com/en/do-work) where she demonstrates the process with actual clients.

How to Create Healthy Changes that Last

Step two in your Hormone Harmony Action Plan is to tackle habit changes. If you know you're in perimenopause (or if you scored greater than three on my quiz), it's time to get busy. Habit change is hard. I work a lot on goal-setting and accountability with my clients. I think it's one of the most important services I offer because left to their own devices without support, most of my clients will revert back to old habits despite good intentions. In the years I've been doing this work, I've found the following things to be critical when it comes to implementing healthy changes.

Focus on one goal at a time

Most of us think we're great at multi-tasking, but studies have shown again and again that this is not true. The same is true for habit change. It is very difficult to take on multiple goals or areas of focus at once. Savvy Sisters know that "eating the elephant" one bite a time is the recipe for success.

Let's say you have five goals you want to achieve. Pick one to focus on first. I often recommend to first set up momentum for success. Break your first goal into mini-steps that feel easily doable. Then take it one step at a time. Keep doing this until the goal is accomplished. Then, when your first goal is completed, move to the next one.

Eliminate the non-essential

First, identify the essential things in your life that are most important to you (no more than five). These are your absolute yesses. Then eliminate everything else from your priority list. This simplifies things and leaves you with the space to focus on what is really important to you. This process works with anything—your life in general or work projects and tasks. Clearing the clutter of "busyness" leaves space for you.

Create a daily routine

Most of us live our days in reactive mode. That means from the time our eyes open in the morning we are not consciously choosing how we spend our energy. Instead, we react to whatever is making the most noise in our lives. Creating a daily routine for yourself can make a big difference in your life and help you to feel more grounded all day. The best routines bookmark the beginning and end of the day both for your workday and for your day in general. Here's what this might look like:

- Wake up and exercise, meditate, or read something inspirational, then eat breakfast.
- Go to your office, take a few deep breaths, then choose your two main priorities for the day.
- At the end of your work day, straighten your desk, shut down your computer, and walk away.
- In your evening time, you may want to meditate again or light candles and read a book before bed.

It doesn't really matter what you choose as long as whatever you choose helps you feel grounded. These lines of demarcation in your day help your brain transition from personal to work time and back again.

Detox your life beyond your body and busyness

Now's the time to evaluate relationships (family and friends), work responsibilities, your environment, etc., and determine if any of these areas are causing you undue stress. You are not required to hang onto people and/or things that no longer serve you or bring you joy. This is an absolutely critical component of stress management because things and/or people that bring you down will derail you faster than you can say "boo!"

Lastly, get accountability

Whether it's hiring a coach or finding a friend or group to be your cheerleader and keep your feet to the fire, accountability is powerful. When you tell another person the action steps you plan to implement, the likelihood is much higher that you will do what you say you'll do.

Get Help to Nourish Your Body

Step three of your Hormone Harmony Action Plan is to consider where your body might need additional support with supplements or vitamins. As you've been reading this book, I hope you've jotted down anything that sounds like it will benefit you. If not, look back at my Foundational Five in the chapter on supplements and start there. This may also be the step where you want to consider hormone testing to see where your imbalances lie so they can be addressed directly. I recommend getting professional help with this. The number of women who insist on taking a do-it-yourself approach to hormone management is stunning to me. Would you treat your own diabetes or heart disease? If not, why would you approach hormones differently? You will definitely get further faster by working with an expert.

Continue Your Learning

Step four is to educate yourself about menopause. You're probably shaking your head thinking that this book would be all you'd ever need to know. Nope. Savvy Sisters need to know what happens when your ovaries retire for good, periods stop, and hormones hit rock bottom. Low estrogen and low testosterone bring on different symptoms and require different approaches to management. Menopausal women also need to know how to protect bone, skin, brain, and heart health as they age, as well as the benefits and risks of hormone replacement therapy. Now is the time to learn about these things so you'll be prepared to talk with your health care team about what you want for your health. You are in charge of it 24/7. I've listed some credible websites for you to begin learning about menopause in the Resources chapter.

Looking Ahead

Let me leave you with this. Imagine the day has finally arrived when you've achieved hormonal balance (cue the choir of angels). You are exercising most days in ways that feel like love to your body. You're sleeping a solid eight hours a night. Sugar doesn't really taste good anymore. You feel healthy and more alive than you have in a long time. Drudgery has turned to delight, and you worry so much less about your health.

Don't look back. You're now armed with the tools you need to create a plan and sustain the changes you make. But here's one more thing to know. There will be moments when you backslide. This is perfectly normal, and it offers you an opportunity to reaffirm the importance of putting yourself first. What causes this backsliding to happen? In my experience it is almost always stress. You get busy and stressed out, which leads to mindless behaviors. What's the solution? Don't take your eye off the prize. Step back, take some deep breaths, and refocus.

My wish for you is that you take what I've written here and put together your own prescription to feel savvy, sane, and sparkly from the inside out. You can download a free copy of my Hormony Harmony Action Plan template at www.drannagarrett.com. You deserve a life that's full of joy, confidence, and happiness, and that life is absolutely possible. You deserve to feel at home in your skin again. Celebrate the victories, large and small. And remember, achieving hormone balance is a process and takes time. Be kind to yourself on your journey.

You've got this!

Acknowledgements

Writing a book is hard work, and it takes a village to get to the point where you are holding your "baby" in your hands. I'd first like to acknowledge the ladies of the Hormone Harmony Club. Without your bravery and your stories, there would have been no inspiration to put my "ass in chair" for the amount of sitting-still time this took to complete. Thanks for cheering me on in the background! I appreciate you all more than you know.

To Lisa Larter and the ladies at the Beach House Mastermind, thanks for the kick in the pants I needed to set this as my 2018 goal and to begin.

To Tammy Plunkett, my writing coach, who lovingly prodded me on, one chapter at a time, every two weeks. I would never have had the discipline to do this myself. And I appreciate that you have a team of expert editors and distributors who made the process of getting this out in the world seamless for me.

And finally, to my husband, Dan. I know I missed a lot of hikes and hanging out together because of this. Thank you for your support and patience, and for allowing me the quiet time and space to get my thoughts on paper. I appreciate it, and I love you!

Resources

There are many resources for women in perimenopause, some of which are more reliable than others. Here, I have curated a list of resources I find credible and helpful.

Practitioners

As a certified coach, hormone expert, and Doctor of Pharmacy, I help busy professional women who are sick and tired of being sick and tired get their hormones back in balance, so they can live happy, healthy, productive lives. I also consult with corporations and other organizations who want to create a culture of empathy and compassion for midlife women.

Take my perimenopause quiz to find out if it's likely that you're experiencing perimenopause. Find it at www.perimenopausequiz.com.
My web address is www.drannagarrett.com.

Dr. Sara Gottfried's mission at the Gottfried Institute—and in life—is to help people feel vital and

balanced from their cells to their souls. She is the author of *The Hormone Cure*, *The Hormone Cure Diet*, and *Younger: A Breakthrough Program to Reset Your Genes, Reverse Aging, and Turn Back the Clock 10 Years.*
www.saragottfried.com

Dr. Josh Axe, DC, DNM, CNS, is a Doctor of Chiropractic, certified doctor of natural medicine, and clinical nutritionist with a passion for helping people to eat healthy and live a healthy lifestyle. In 2008, he started a functional medicine center in Nashville, which has grown to become one of the most renowned clinics in the world.
www.draxe.com

Marcelle Pick, NP, is passionate about transforming the way women experience healthcare through an integrative approach. She co-founded the world-renowned Women to Women Clinic in 1983 with a vision of not only treating illness, but also helping support her patients to proactively make healthier choices to prevent disease.
www.marcellepick.com

Christiane Northrup, MD, is a visionary pioneer and a leading authority in the field of women's health and wellness, which includes the unity of mind, body, emotions, and spirit. Internationally known for her empowering approach to women's health and wellness, Dr. Northrup teaches women how to thrive at every stage of life.
www.drnorthrup.com

This the official website of the North American Menopause Society. While I don't always agree with their positions on issues, there is a lot of good, evidence-based info here.
www.menopause.org

Supplements

Quality matters! You can find the products I recommend in the book through the link below. Wellevate stocks only top-quality supplements that I trust for my clients' health.
www.wellevate.me/drannagarrett

Lab Tests

If you live near a Quest blood draw center, you can order your own blood work for much less than what you'll pay through insurance. Use the link below to search for labs or contact me for guidance. I offer interpretation of lab results for a consultation fee.
www.ultalabtests.com/drannagarrett

Direct-to-consumer saliva hormone testing and dried urine hormone testing are available in the U.S. from the following companies:
ZRT Labs: www.zrtlab.com
Precision Analytical: www.dutchtest.com

Facebook Groups

Hormone Harmony Club

www.drannagarrett.com/hhc
This is my free, private group on Facebook. It is moderated by community members, and I pop in now and then to say hello. The purpose is to support women and share information. We do not answer specific medical questions or interpret lab results.

Dr. Anna's Savvy, Sane Sisterhood

www.facebook.com/groups/savvysanesisterhood/
This is the private Facebook group for paid members of the Savvy Sane Sisterhood. This is a membership group I created for women who want more of my help with education and hormone management. We have monthly question and answer calls, expert Deep Dive calls in areas of interest to women in midlife, a private Facebook group just for the Sisterhood. You can find out more about that here:
www.drannagarrett.com/savvy-sane-sisterhood.

Menopause Chicks

www.facebook.com/groups/MenopauseChicks/
Menopause Chicks empowers women to navigate perimenopause and menopause with confidence and ease. My friend, Shirley Weir (creator of the group), does this by connecting women to the best information and the top women's health professionals who can support them on their journey.

Midlife and Menopause Solutions

www.facebook.com/groups/midlifemenopausesoluti
ons/
This group is the place to come to ask questions, give advice, share stories, rant, rave, laugh, and learn. In this group, we believe our midlife (and beyond!) years can and should be the best years of our lives, and we're here to help make it happen for all women.

Healthy Eating

Dani Spies is a powerhouse of knowledge when it comes to clean eating, and she offers amazing recipes on her site (try the simmered turkey meatballs). She has a great YouTube channel. You definitely want to check her out if you need help with your eating habits or you'd like recipe ideas.
www.cleananddelicious.com
www.youtube.com/user/danispies

Mental Health

Canada

www.suicideprevention.ca

U.S.

National Suicide Prevention Lifeline 800-273-8255
www.suicidepreventionlifeline.org

UK

www.samaritans.org
116 123 (UK)
116 123 (ROI)
www.mind.org.uk
0300 123 3393 or text 86463

Notes

Chapter 1

34 menopause symptoms. www.34-menopause-symptoms.com/. Accessed December 10, 2018.

Chapter 2

Turner N. The most common hormonal imbalances and how to recognize if it's a problem for you. The Marilyn Dennis Show. May 2, 2012. https://www.marilyn.ca/Health/Articles/May-2012/Most_recognized_hormonal_imbalances. Accessed December 13, 2018.

Facts about DIM and women's health. World Health Botanicals. https://wholeworldbotanicals.com/facts-about-dim-and-womens-health/. Accessed December 13, 2018.

Glycemic index and diabetes. www.diabetes.org/food-and-fitness/food/what-can-i-eat/understanding-carbohydrates/glycemic-index-and-diabetes.html. Accessed December 10,2018.

Virgin JJ. 5 Reasons intermittent fasting could become a bad idea. www.huffpost.com/entry/intermittent-fasting_b_5541429. September 8, 2014. Accessed December 6, 2018

Link R. Paleo Diet Plan, Best Paleo Foods + Paleo Diet Recipes. Dr. Axe. December 3, 2017. draxe.com. https://www.draxe.com/paleo-diet-plan/. Accessed December 13, 2018.

10 low glycemic foods that help burn fat. Healthy Holistic Living. healthy-holistic-living.com. https://www.healthy-holistic-living.com/low-glycemic-foods.html. Accessed December 15, 2018.

Chapter 3

Ferrie JE,Shipley MJ, Cappuccio FP et al. A Prospective Study of Change in Sleep Duration: Associations with Mortality in the Whitehall II Cohort. Sleep 2007 Dec 1; 30(12): 1659–1666.

Hong KB, Park Y, Suh HJ. Sleep-promoting effects of the GABA/5-HTP mixture in vertebrate models. Behav Brain Res. 2016 Sep 1;310:36-41.

Lindahl O, Lindwall L.Double blind study of a valerian preparation. Pharmacol Biochem Behav. 1989 Apr;32(4):1065-6.

Cases J, Ibarra A Feuillère N eta al. Pilot trial of *Melissa officinalis* L. leaf extract in the treatment of volunteers suffering from mild-to-moderate anxiety disorders and sleep disturbances. Med J Nutrition Metab. 2011 Dec; 4(3): 211–218

Chapter 4

Livdans-Forret AB, Harvey PJ, Larkin-Their SM. Menorrhagia: A synopsis of management focusing on herbal and nutritional supplements, and chiropractic. J Can Chiropr Assoc. 2007 Dec; 51(4): 235–246. Cook M. "Hormonal contraception boosts risk for breast cancer in Danish study." Bioedge.org. December 9, 2017. https://www.bioedge.org/bioethics/hormonal-contraception-boosts-risk-for-breast-cancer-in-danish-study/12546. Accessed December 15, 2018.

Northrup, C. Heavy menstrual bleeding (menorrhagia). Drnorthrup.com. https://www.drnorthrup.com/heavy-menstrual-bleeding-menorrhagia/. Accessed December 15, 2018.

Chapter 5

U.S. suicide rates are rising faster among women than men. NPR.org. June 14, 2018 www.npr.org/sections/health-shots/2018/06/14/619338703/u-s-suicides-rates-are-rising-faster-among-women-than-men. Accessed December 10, 2018.

Study reveals 70% of women in perimenopause lack adequate support network. Newswire.ca. October 30, 2017. https://www.newswire.ca/news-releases/study-reveals-70-of-women-in-perimenopause-lack-adequate-support-network-654057843.html?fbclid=IwAR1EIPpgeiJZ-bRtXXQ7KSHc2Sl2gyqVaKr51BDWRlGWKmqk-Zw986FMP9E. Accessed December 12, 2018.

Pratte MA, Nanavati KB, Young V et al. An Alternative Treatment for Anxiety: A Systematic Review of Human Trial Results Reported for the Ayurvedic Herb Ashwagandha (*Withania somnifera*). J Altern Complement Med. 2014 Dec 1; 20(12): 901–908.

Sarris J, Stough C, Bousman CA, et al. Kava in the treatment of generalized anxiety disorder: a double-blind, randomized, placebo-controlled study. J Clin Psychopharmacol. 2013 Oct;33(5):643-8

Kasper S, Gastpar M, Müller WE, et al. Silexan, an orally administered Lavandula oil preparation, is effective in the treatment of 'subsyndromal' anxiety disorder: a randomized, double-blind, placebo-controlled trial. *Int Clin Psychopharmacol* 2010. Sep;25(5):277-87.

Symptoms. Anxiety and Depression Association of America. adaa.org. https://adaa.org/understanding-anxiety/panic-disorder-agoraphobia/symptoms. Accessed December 15, 2018.

Natural depression treatment. drweil.com. https://www.drweil.com/health-wellness/body-mind-

spirit/mental-health/natural-depression-treatment/.
Accessed December 15, 2018.

Chapter 6

Basaraba S. How Smoking Causes Early Aging and
Premature Wrinkles. Very Well Mind. June 14,
2018. https://www.verywellmind.com/how-smoking-
ages-skin-2223424. Accessed December 15, 2018.

Emiling S. Sleep deprivation linked to aging skin,
study suggests. Huffington Post. July 24,
2013.huffingtonpost.com.
https://www.huffingtonpost.com/2013/07/24/sleep-
deprivation-effects-aging-skin_n_3644269.html. Accessed December 15, 2018.

Seidman A. Sitting for more than three hours a day
cuts life expectancy.
www.wsj.com/articles/SB10001424052702303343 4
04577516853567934264. July 10, 2012. Accessed
December 11, 2018.

van der Ploeg HP, Chey T, Korda RJ, et al. Sitting
time and all-cause mortality risk in 222 497 Australian adults. Arch Intern Med. 2012;172(6):494-500.

Tarkan, L. The connection between sitting and diabetes
www.ontrackdiabetes.com/get-
fit/motivation/connection-between-sitting-diabetes
July 27, 2017. Accessed December 11, 2018.

Brehony KA. *Awakening at Midlife: A Guide to Reviving Your Spirit, Recreating Your Life, and Returning to Your Truest Self.* Riverhead Books; 1997.

Chapter 7

Menopause transition: effects on women's economic participation. https://www.gov.uk/government/publications/menopause-transition-effects-on-womens-economic-participation. July 20, 2017. Accessed December 11, 2018.

Berlinsky-Schine R. Menopause age: when it happens and how to manage it at work. www.fairygodboss.com/career-topics/menopause-age-and-the-workplace-keeping-menopause-from-interfering. Accessed December 6, 2018.

Newson LR. Menopause discrimination is a real thing and bosses need to get involved. Telegraph.co.uk. October 18, 2017. https://www.telegraph.co.uk/women/work/menopause-discrimination-real-thing-bosses-need-get-involved/. Accessed December 16, 2018.

Martin JA, Hamilton BE, Osterman MJK. Births in the United States, 2017. NCHS Data Brief, Number 318; August 2018. www.cdc.gov/nchs/data/databriefs/..Accessed December 6, 2018.

Stoppler MC. Puberty.
https://www.medicinenet.com/puberty/article.htm.
May 7, 2018. Accessed December 12, 2018.

Chapter 8

The effects of stress on your
body.www.webmd.com/balance/stress-
management/effects-of-stress-on-your-body.

Weaver J. Can stress actually be good for you?
http://www.nbcnews.com/id/15818153/ns/health-
mental_health/t/can-stress-actually-be-good-you/ -
.W_12lpNKh98. December 20, 2006. Accessed December 12, 2018.

McEvoy M.Cortisol and DHEA: the major hormone
balance. Metabolic Healing.
metabolichealing.com.
https://metabolichealing.com/cortisol-dhea-the-
major-hormone-balance/. Accessed December 16,
2018.

Chandrasekhar K, Kapoor J, Sridhar A. A Prospective, Randomized Double-Blind, Placebo-Controlled
Study of Safety and Efficacy of a High-
Concentration Full-Spectrum Extract of
Ashwagandha Root in Reducing Stress and Anxiety
in Adults. Indian J Psychol Med. 2012 Jul-Sep;
34(3): 255–262. Accessed December 6, 2018.

Ishaque S, Shamseer L, Bukutu C, et al. *Rhodiola
rosea* for physical and mental fatigue: a systematic

review. BMC Complement Altern Med. Published online 2012 May 29. doi: [10.1186/1472-6882-12-70]. Accessed December 6, 2018

Summary of bacopa monnieri. https://examine.com/supplements/bacopa-monnieri/. October 9, 2018. Accessed December 6, 2018.
.
Conforth T. Chasteberry for treatment of menstrual problems. https://www.verywellhealth.com/what-is-chasteberry-2721967. May 27, 2018. Accessed December 12, 2018.

Chapter 9

Brodwin E. The $37 billion supplement industry is barely regulated—and it's allowing dangerous products to slip through the cracks. Business Insider. November 8, 2017. https://www.businessinsider.com/supplements-vitamins-bad-or-good-health-2017-8. Accessed December 16, 2018.

Boost magnesium levels to rebalance your hormones. Hormones and Balance. https://hormonesbalance.com/articles/boost-magnesium-levels-to-rebalance-your-hormones/. Accessed December 16, 2018.

Neuzil A. Ask the ND: The Best Kind of Magnesium For You. Peoplesrx. http://www.peoplesrx.com/the-best-kind-of-magnesium-for-you/. Accessed December 16, 2018.

Conforth T. Chasteberry for treatment of menstrual problems. http://www.verywellhealth.com/what-is-chasteberry-2721967. May 27, 2018. Accessed December 12, 2018.

Chapter 10

Wolff J. What doctors don't know about menopause. www.aarp.org/health/conditionstreatments/info-2018/menopause-symptoms-doctors-relief-treatment.html. August/September 2108. Accessed December 12, 2018.

Chapter 11

To Remove the Cervix or Preserve It During Hysterectomy? Your Options Explained. MIS for Women. August 12, 2014.misforwomen.com. http://www.misforwomen.com/to-remove-the-cervix-or-preserve-it-during-hysterectomy-your-options-explained/. Accessed December 17, 2018.

Types of hysterectomy. http://www.healthcommunities.com/gynecologic-surgery/types-surgical-procedures-hysterectomy.html. September 17, 2015. Accessed December 12, 2018.

Brown JJ. 10 Things Your Doctor Won't Tell You About Hysterectomy. Everyday Health everydayhealth.com. https://www.everydayhealth.com/news/things-your-doctor-wont-tell-you-about-hysterectomy/. Accessed December 17, 2018.

Hysterectomies that save ovaries still carry health risks, study finds.
https://www.cleveland.com/healthfit/index.ssf/2018/02/hysterectomies_that_save_ovari.html. February 8, 2018. Accessed December 12, 2018.

Index